Neuropsychiatric Assessment

Review of Psychiatry Series
John M. Oldham, M.D., M.S.
Michelle B. Riba, M.D., M.S.
Series Editors

Neuropsychiatric Assessment

EDITED BY

Stuart C. Yudofsky, M.D.

H. Florence Kim, M.D.

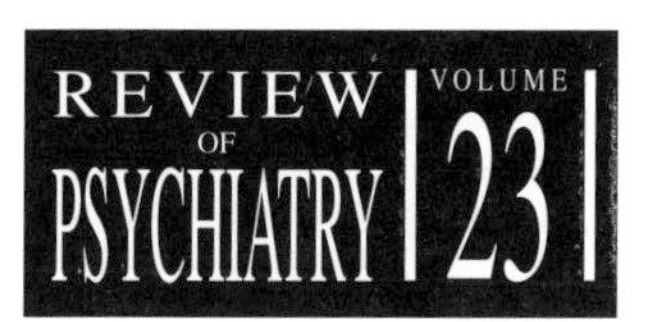

No. 2

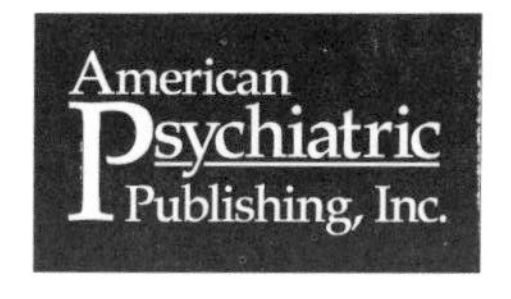

Washington, DC
London, England

Note: The authors have worked to ensure that all information in this book is accurate at the time of publication and consistent with general psychiatric and medical standards, and that information concerning drug dosages, schedules, and routes of administration is accurate at the time of publication and consistent with standards set by the U.S. Food and Drug Administration and the general medical community. As medical research and practice continue to advance, however, therapeutic standards may change. Moreover, specific situations may require a specific therapeutic response not included in this book. For these reasons and because human and mechanical errors sometimes occur, we recommend that readers follow the advice of physicians directly involved in their care or the care of a member of their family.

Manufactured in the United States of America on acid-free paper
08 07 06 05 04 5 4 3 2 1
First Edition

Typeset in Adobe's Palatino

American Psychiatric Publishing, Inc.
1000 Wilson Boulevard
Arlington, VA 22209-3901
www.appi.org

The correct citation for this book is
Yudofsky SC, Kim HF (editors): *Neuropsychiatric Assessment* (Review of Psychiatry Series, Volume 23; Oldham JM and Riba MB, series editors). Washington, DC, American Psychiatric Publishing, 2004

Library of Congress Cataloging-in-Publication Data
Neuropsychiatric Assessment / edited by Stuart C. Yudofsky, H. Florence Kim.
— 1st ed.
p. ; cm. — (Review of psychiatry, ISSN 1041-5882 ; v. 23, no. 2)
Includes bibliographical references and index.
ISBN 1-58562-177-3 (pbk. : alk. paper)
1. Mental illness—Diagnosis. 2. Nervous system—Diseases—Diagnosis.
3. Neuropsychological tests. 4. Neuropsychiatry. I. Yudofsky, Stuart C.
II. Kim, H. Florence, 1971–. III. Review of psychiatry series ; v. 23, 2.
[DNLM: 1. Mental disorders—diagnosis. 2. Neuropsychological Tests.
3. Diagnostic Imaging—methods. 4. Nervous System Diseases—diagnosis.
5. Neuropsychology—methods. WM 145.5.N4 N494 2004]
RC473.N48N466 2004
616.89'075—dc22 2003065581

British Library Cataloguing in Publication Data
A CIP record is available from the British Library.

Contents

Contributors

Nashaat N. Boutros, M.D.
Associate Professor of Psychiatry, Yale University School of Medicine, New Haven, Connecticut; VA Connecticut Healthcare System, West Haven, Connecticut

Glen E. Getz, M.A.
Doctoral Candidate, University of Cincinnati, Department of Clinical Psychology, Cincinnati, Ohio; Clinical Psychology Intern, Allegheny General Hospital, Department of Psychiatry, Pittsburgh, Pennsylvania

H. Florence Kim, M.D.
Assistant Professor and Medical Director, Neuropsychiatry Programs, Menninger Department of Psychiatry and Behavioral Sciences, Baylor College of Medicine, Houston, Texas

Mark R. Lovell, Ph.D.
Director, University of Pittsburgh School of Medicine, Sports Medicine Concussion Program, Pittsburgh, Pennsylvania

Thomas E. Nordahl, M.D., Ph.D.
Professor, Department of Psychiatry and Behavioral Sciences, University of California, Davis Medical Center, Sacramento, California

John M. Oldham, M.D., M.S.
Professor and Chair, Department of Psychiatry and Behavioral Sciences, Medical University of South Carolina, Charleston, South Carolina

Fred Ovsiew, M.D.
Professor of Psychiatry; Chief, Clinical Neuropsychiatry; Medical Director, Adult Inpatient Psychiatry, Department of Psychiatry, University of Chicago Hospitals, Chicago, Illinois

Michelle B. Riba, M.D., M.S.
Clinical Professor and Associate Chair for Education and Academic Affairs, Department of Psychiatry, University of Michigan Medical School, Ann Arbor, Michigan

Ruth Salo, Ph.D.
Assistant Research Neuropsychologist, Department of Psychiatry and Behavioral Sciences, University of California, Davis Medical Center, Sacramento, California

Frederick A. Struve, Ph.D.
Senior Research Scientist, Yale University School of Medicine, New Haven, Connecticut

Stuart C. Yudofsky, M.D.
The D.C. and Irene Ellwood Chair of Psychiatry and Chairman and Professor, Menninger Department of Psychiatry and Behavioral Sciences, Baylor College of Medicine, Houston, Texas; Chief of Psychiatry Service, The Methodist Hospital, Houston, Texas

Introduction to the Review of Psychiatry Series

John M. Oldham, M.D., M.S.
Michelle B. Riba, M.D., M.S., Series Editors

2004 Review of Psychiatry Series Titles

- *Developmental Psychobiology*
  Edited by B.J. Casey, Ph.D.
- *Neuropsychiatric Assessment*
  Edited by Stuart C. Yudofsky, M.D., and H. Florence Kim, M.D.
- *Brain Stimulation in Psychiatric Treatment*
  Edited by Sarah H. Lisanby, M.D.
- *Cognitive-Behavior Therapy*
  Edited by Jesse H. Wright, M.D., Ph.D.

Throughout the country, media coverage is responding to increased popular demand for information about the brain—what it does, how it works, and what to expect of it throughout the life cycle. For example, in a special issue of *Scientific American* called "Better Brains: How Neuroscience Will Enhance You," in September 2003, leading researchers summarized exciting new frontiers in psychiatry, including neuroplasticity, new diagnostic technology, new drug development informed by knowledge about gene sequences and molecular configurations, new directions in stress management guided by increased understanding of the effects of stress on the brain, and brain stimulation techniques related to the revolutionary recognition that neurogenesis can occur in the adult brain. This special issue illustrates the enormous excitement about developments in brain science.

In our scientific journals, there is an explosion of information about neuroscience and about the bidirectional nature of brain and behavior. The matter was previously debated as if one had to choose between two camps (mind versus brain), but a rapidly developing new paradigm is replacing this former dichotomy—that the brain influences behavior, and that the mind (ideas, emotions, hopes, aspirations, anxieties, fears, and the wide realm of real and perceived environmental experience) influences the brain. The term *neuropsychiatry* has served as successor to the former term *organic psychiatry* and is contrasted with notions of psychodynamics, such as the concept of unconsciously motivated behavior. As our field evolves and matures, we are developing a new language for meaningful but imperfectly understood earlier concepts. *Subliminal cues* and *indirect memory* are among the terms of our new language, but the emerging understanding that experience itself can activate genes and stimulate protein synthesis, cellular growth, and neurogenesis is a groundbreaking new synthesis of concepts that previously seemed incompatible. Among the remarkable conclusions that these new findings suggest is that psychotherapy can be construed as a biological treatment, in the sense that it has the potential to alter the cellular microanatomy of the brain.

In the context of this rapidly changing scientific and clinical landscape, we selected for the 2004 Review of Psychiatry four broad areas of attention: 1) research findings in developmental psychobiology, 2) current recommendations for neuropsychiatric assessment of patients, 3) new treatments in the form of brain stimulation techniques, and 4) the application of cognitive-behavior therapy as a component of treatment of patients with severely disabling psychiatric disorders.

Perhaps the logical starting place in the 2004 series is *Developmental Psychobiology*, edited by B.J. Casey. Derived from research that uses animal models and studies of early human development, this work summarizes the profound impact of early environmental events. Following a comprehensive overview of the field by Casey, elegant studies of the developmental psychobiology of attachment are presented by Hofer, one of the pioneers in this work. Specific areas of research are then described in detail: the developmental neurobiology of an early maturational task called face processing (Scott and Nelson); findings in the developmental psychobiology of reading disability (McCandliss and Wolmetz); current thinking about the central relevance of early development in the disabling condition Gilles de la Tourette's syndrome (Gallardo, Swain, and Leckman); and the early development of the prefrontal cortex and the implications of these findings in adult-onset schizophrenia (Erickson and Lewis).

Stuart C. Yudofsky and H. Florence Kim, the editors of *Neuropsychiatric Assessment,* have gathered together experts to bring us up to date on the current practice of neuropsychiatric physical diagnosis (Ovsiew); the importance of the neuropsychological examination of psychiatric patients (Getz and Lovell); and the use of electrophysiological testing (Boutros and Struve) and neuropsychiatric laboratory testing (Kim and Yudofsky) in clinical practice. Any focus on neuropsychiatry today must include information about developments in brain imaging; here the clinical usefulness of selected neuroimaging techniques for specific psychiatric disorders is reviewed by Nordahl and Salo.

A particularly interesting area of clinical research, and one with promising potential to provide new treatment techniques, is that of stimulating the brain. The long-known phenomenon of "magnetism" has emerged in a fascinating new incarnation, referred to in its central nervous system applications as transcranial magnetic stimulation (TMS). Sarah H. Lisanby edited *Brain Stimulation in Psychiatric Treatment,* in which TMS is described in connection with its possible use in depression (Schlaepfer and Kosel) and in schizophrenia and other disorders (Hoffman). New applications in psychiatry of deep brain stimulation, a technique showing great promise in Parkinson's disease and other neurological conditions, are reviewed (Greenberg), and the current state of knowledge about magnetic seizure therapy (Lisanby) and vagal nerve stimulation (Sackeim) is presented. All of these roads of investigation have the potential to lead to new, perhaps more effective treatments for our patients.

Finally, in *Cognitive-Behavior Therapy,* edited by Jesse H. Wright, the broadening scope of cognitive therapy is considered with regard to schizophrenia (Scott, Kingdon, and Turkington), bipolar disorder (Basco, McDonald, Merlock, and Rush), medical patients (Sensky), and children and adolescents (Albano, Krain, Podniesinksi, and Ditkowsky). Technological advances in the form of computer-assisted cognitive behavior therapy are presented as well (Wright).

All in all, in our view the selected topics for 2004 represent a rich sampling of the amazing developments taking place in brain science and psychiatric evaluation and treatment. We believe that we have put together an equally relevant menu for 2005, when the Review of Psychiatry Series will include volumes on psychiatric genetics (Kenneth Kendler, editor); sleep disorders and psychiatry (Daniel Buysse, editor); pregnancy and postpartum depression (Lee Cohen, editor); and bipolar disorder (Terence Ketter, Charles Bowden, and Joseph Calabrese, editors).

Introduction

Stuart C. Yudofsky, M.D.
H. Florence Kim, M.D.

What is neuropsychiatry? Neuropsychiatry is an integrative and collaborative field that brings together brain and behavior. Yudofsky and Hales (1989) described the underlying tenets of the discipline to be the "inseparability of brain and thought, of mind and body, and of mental and physical" (p. 1). Neuropsychiatry attempts to bridge the artificial boundaries between neurology and psychiatry in order to treat the multitude of clinical manifestations of the singular brain. Neuropsychiatry is primarily focused on the assessment and treatment of the cognitive, behavioral, and mood symptoms of patients with neurological disorders. However, an equally important focus for neuropsychiatrists is the understanding of the role of brain dysfunction in the pathogenesis of primary psychiatric disorders (Yudofsky and Hales 2002). Therefore, not only does neuropsychiatry bring the psychiatric assessment and treatment of psychotic or mood symptoms to the neurology arena, it also returns clinicians to the objective rigors of physical diagnosis and testing, which are often not practiced in psychiatry today.

This volume in the Review of Psychiatry Series provides an overview of the neuropsychiatric approach to assessment and presents discussions of techniques and testing methods that may be more familiar to neurologists than to psychiatrists. However, all these techniques have clinical applications for the psychiatric patient and are presented with this focus in mind.

The cornerstone of any neuropsychiatric assessment is the physical examination and the medical and psychiatric history. Fred Ovsiew, M.D., provides a masterful overview of the bedside neuropsychiatric examination and details ways to obtain a history tailored to common neuropsychiatric complaints. He provides a head-to-toe compendium of important signs and symptoms to be elicited and presents the differential diagnoses of neuropsychiatric disorders that should be entertained when faced with a particular constellation of signs and symptoms.

The physical examination is indeed an underappreciated and underutilized entity in modern psychiatry, and Dr. Ovsiew skillfully illustrates how essential it is to the neuropsychiatric approach.

Another essential component of the neuropsychiatric assessment is the neuropsychological examination. Neuropsychological and psychological measures are often overlooked in the routine workup of psychiatric patients, because these instruments are generally administered by neuropsychologists. Glen E. Getz, M.A., and Mark Lovell, Ph.D., illustrate the utility of the neuropsychological examination in the assessment of the neuropsychiatric patient. They discuss the clinical approach to the interview process, fixed-battery and flexible-battery approaches to neuropsychological assessment, and pitfalls encountered during the interpretation of test results, and future trends in neuropsychological assessment. They emphasize the major cognitive domains that may be involved in neuropsychiatric disorders and explain how a specific pattern of deficits in certain domains may help to determine a neuropsychiatric diagnosis.

Electrophysiological testing is an underutilized modality in psychiatry, but it is invaluable for the diagnosis and evaluation of some neuropsychiatric disorders. Nashaat N. Boutros, M.D., and Frederick S. Struve, Ph.D., provide an introduction to standard electroencephalography, cerebral evoked potentials, topographic quantitative electroencephalography, and polysomnography and explain the relevance of these testing modalities to neuropsychiatric disorders. They also provide recommendations for electrophysiological testing in certain clinical situations, such as behavioral disturbance, cognitive decline, rapid-cycling bipolar disorder, and panic disorder and outline the possible broader uses of electrophysiological testing in neuropsychiatry in the future.

Laboratory testing and neuroimaging are more commonly used modalities in neuropsychiatry. They are particularly important to the neuropsychiatric approach because of the complex array of neurological and medical illnesses that may underlie the psychiatric symptoms of the neuropsychiatric patient. H. Florence Kim, M.D., and Stuart C. Yudofsky, M.D., discuss the current lack of consensus guidelines for screening psychiatric patients with conventional laboratory testing, chest radiography, and electrocardiography as well as the more extensive workup that may be necessary for a patient with neuropsychiatric symptoms.

Perhaps the modality that is most synonymous with the neuropsychiatric approach is neuroimaging. The popularity of neuropsychiatry has been augmented by new and ever more sophisticated neuroimaging approaches that have been developed over the past 30 years that allow psychiatrists to see the brain and its pathways with a clarity once unimaginable. Thomas E. Nordahl, M.D., Ph.D., and Ruth Salo, Ph.D., discuss several of these modalities, including structural and functional magnetic resonance imaging, magnetic resonance spectroscopy, diffusion tensor imaging, and positron emission tomography. They provide a fascinating overview of the techniques involved as well as the current research findings with these modalities in patients with schizophrenia, major affective disorder, and obsessive-compulsive disorder.

References

Yudofsky SC, Hales RE: The reemergence of neuropsychiatry: definition and direction. J Neuropsychiatry Clin Neurosci 1:1–6, 1989

Yudofsky SC, Hales RE: Neuropsychiatry and the future of psychiatry and neurology. Am J Psychiatry 159:1261–1264, 2002

Chapter 1

Neuropsychiatric Physical Diagnosis in Context

Fred Ovsiew, M.D.

> The first and always most important method of examination is that of conversation with the patient.... A physical examination is of course obligatory in all cases though it only rarely yields results which materially assist the assessment of the mental illness, e.g., in organic cerebral disorders and the symptomatic psychoses.
>
> *Jaspers (1963), pp. 826–827*

The above excerpt from Jaspers's (1963) *General Psychopathology*—correctly taken to represent the best of the descriptive psychiatric tradition—is echoed in contemporary psychiatric texts. The physical examination is "obligatory," and, naturally, what a person is obliged to do has been considered work and has been shunned, in practice even if never in theory. Perhaps the aversion has extended from the physical examination to any focused medical inquiry. This chapter focuses on some of these specialized tools, partly to redress what appears to be an imbalance in the current state of psychiatric practice, in which conversation has vanquished the medical examination. In view of the solid evidence for the high prevalence of organic contributors to psychopathology in many clinical populations (Yates and Koran 1999), a reemphasis on medical assessment is appropriate.

The crucial cognitive and mental state examinations are discussed widely elsewhere, including other chapters in this volume (Lishman 1998; Ovsiew 2002; Ovsiew and Bylsma 2002). By contrast, guidance for the neuropsychiatric physical examination is rarely provided in textbooks, although of course superb general texts on the physical examination are available (McGee 2001; Orient and Sapira 2000). For example, in *Psychiatry* Tasman et al. (1997) offer this advice, *tout court:* "All patients presenting with 'psychiatric' symptoms require a careful and complete physical examination" (p. 540). Similarly, Andreasen and Black (2001) make the following suggestion: "The general physical examination should follow the standard format used in the rest of medicine, covering organ systems of the body from head to foot.... Likewise, a standard neurological examination should be done" (p. 57). All examiners should be careful, but no examiner can be complete "from head to foot." Just as an endocrinologist's physical examination will focus on the findings relevant to endocrine disease, the physician in psychological medicine should know what to give priority to in taking a history and performing a physical examination, while keeping an eye open for a surprise. Priorities should be based on a sound grasp of the psychopathology of organic disease and evolving hypotheses about the patient's illness. In this chapter I explore the general medical history, the general physical examination, and the elementary neurological examination as probes with the capacity to highlight contributions of organic brain disease to mental symptoms. Sanders and Keshavan (2002) provided similar coverage. Findings that are consequent to psychiatric illness or its treatment (for example, a rash caused by psychotropic drugs) or incidental though important (for example, coexisting hypertension in a schizophrenic patient) are not emphasized.

Context

The foundation of the approach elaborated in this chapter is that the bedside neuropsychiatric examination is a naturalistic enterprise, in contrast to methods such as neuroimaging, neuropsychological assessment, and laboratory testing. These methods produce information of inestimable importance, information that should sharpen bedside observational tools. Yet certain information can be gathered only in the consulting room, by history taking and clinical examination. The clinician is in a position to discern phenomena not revealed in other ways.

The privileged access provided by the neuropsychiatric examination includes a view of the patient's subjective experience. The neuropsychiatry of subjective experience is distinct from that of overt behavior. For example, in acute stroke, behavioral manifestations of denial of deficit are distinct from anosognosia, or explicit unawareness of deficit (Ghika-Schmid et al. 1999). Moreover, the anatomical correlates of the two differ as well: anosognosia is linked with a well-known (but inconstant) lateralization to the right hemisphere, whereas denial in behavior is associated with deep lesions in either hemisphere. In general, the anatomical substrates of conscious emotional states (feelings) differ from those of nonconscious emotional processing, specifically in the absence of a role for the amygdala in the former (Dolan 2002).

Furthermore, subjective experience comprises a variety of states that may not lend themselves to analysis in the currently popular framework of modularity. The problem was described beautifully by the neuroanatomist Alf Brodal in his report on his own experience of a stroke, probably a lacuna in the right hemisphere with the clinical picture of pure motor hemiplegia (Brodal 1973). He noted with puzzlement, for example, that despite his being fully dextral his handwriting was altered by a stroke that produced left hemiparesis. He further noted that his concentration had become diminished, that he easily became fatigued with mental work, and that he had loss of automatic movement sequences (such as tying a bow tie: his "fingers did not know the next move"). In summary, he said, "Destruction of even a localized part of the brain will cause consequences for several functions in addition to those which are specifically dependent on the region damaged.... [F]or optimal, perfect, function, we need the whole brain" (p. 688).

By the time of Brodal's self-observations, Teuber and Liebert (1958) had produced a series of experiments delineating the general effects of brain lesions beyond their specific, or localization-related, effects. Chapman and Wolff (1958) and Chapman et al. (1958) had elaborated on the consequences of cerebral damage irrespective of location (but dependent on the volume of tissue lost), describing a reduction in the capacity to recover from stress-produced disruption of performance. This was essentially a version of the "catastrophic reaction" described by Goldstein (1934/1995). For example, if during a timed task a loud noise interfered with the subject's completion of the task, the subjects with brain injury demonstrated a lengthening of the time required to return to the task.

What these authors have proposed is not that subjective experience or personal autonomy exists in a realm divorced from anatomical location or separate from brain mediation. It is that the model of localization may not in all instances perspicuously capture the phenomena of interest. Nor does this proposal argue against continuing attempts to trace the neurobiology of complex mental phenomena (Zysset et al. 2003). Specifically it does not assert that nonlocalized phenomena are socially mediated, although of course social mediation (by stigma, reaction to disability, and so on) cannot be ignored in neuropsychiatric patients. It merely advises that to leave out of consideration phenomena whose localization is poorly understood and for which the assumptions of cerebral modularity may prove inadequate is not a sound way to proceed, either clinically or theoretically. To the contrary, neuropsychiatry is distinctive in a concern for behavioral phenomena that are clearly related to organic disease yet are not related in a simple or (thus far) localizable way. As an example, patients presenting in adulthood with arteriovenous malformations proved to have a history of developmental disturbances in childhood in excess of a comparison population—more reading difficulty, for instance, or more impulsivity, or more problems in drawing or mathematics (Lazar et al. 1999). Yet none of these deficits was associated with the side of the lesion. At present the bedside examination—including history taking and clinical observation—is the most effective way to recognize these general aspects of brain disease, assess their etiology and pathogenesis, and integrate their effects on function into an understanding of the patient.

Why does the neuropsychiatrist need to attend to the patient's subjectivity? Goldstein (1934/1995) argued that symptoms do not directly express damage to the brain but rather reflect the organism's attempt to solve the problems posed by the environment as best it can with reduced resources:

> Symptoms are answers, given by the modified organism, to definite demands; they are attempted solutions to problems derived on the one hand from the demands of the natural environment and on the other from the special tasks imposed on the organism in the course of the examination..... [T]he appearance of symptoms depends on the method of examination. (p. 35)

In similar terms, Syz (1937) wrote:

> Whenever those nervous structures which control the personality-organization are damaged it may become particularly difficult to discriminate between alterations of function due to organic lesions and alterations due to reactive tendencies of the total organism in its adaptation to the environment. So that we may be confronted with combinations or fusions of the two types of processes which are difficult to untangle. (p. 374)

Among the diagnostic tools available to neuropsychiatrists, only the bedside examination is suited to this task. To help the clinician understand not only the disorder, but also more fully the patient who has the disorder, the neuropsychiatric inquiry must find a balance between focused exploration of symptoms and delineation of how those symptoms constrain and determine the patient's experience and functioning.

Taking the Neuropsychiatric History

The clinician pursuing a diagnostic inquiry should obtain a general medical history, specifically as to diseases possibly relevant to the neuropsychiatric symptoms under consideration, and a review of systems in potentially relevant areas. Because a history taken from a psychotic or cognitively impaired patient may be unreliable, collateral informants and review of medical records are commonly essential in neuropsychiatric practice. However, the physician should not overestimate the difficulty of unearthing a medical history. I recall an experience as a psychiatry resident. Having obtained the depression history from my outpatient, I was carefully observing as my attending physician administered the Hamilton Rating Scale for Depression. Relieved of active responsibility for the moment, I regarded my patient with a casual eye—and noticed for the first time the transverse scar on her neck. When the attending physician was finished, I inquired about the scar and learned that the patient had undergone a thyroidectomy. It was then revealed that the patient had stopped taking her thyroid replacement medicine. (It would spoil the story and undercut the moral to add that she proved to be euthyroid.) Such discoveries should be within every physician's ambit and should not be deflected by the psychiatrist to a consultant. Although there is no limit to what medical information might be of importance, Table 1–1 provides a survey of topics that are likely to be pertinent and that should be reviewed with almost every patient. The level of detail of this medical history and of the review of systems should vary according to the clinical context. Positive responses should of course lead to further inquiry. Expertise in eliciting pertinent information about topics of common neuropsychiatric concern will aid in the diagnostic process.

Birth and Early Development

The clinician should explore features of the pregnancy, including maternal substance misuse, bleeding during gestation, and infection. Fetal distress at birth—including Apgar scores if available—and perinatal infection or jaundice should be ascertained. Relevant features of the child's early life include motor and cognitive milestones, such as the ages at which the child crawled, walked, spoke words, and spoke sentences. The infant's school performance (including special education and anomalous profiles of intellectual strengths and weaknesses) is usually the best guide to premorbid intellectual function. In the case of children who have had special education, psychometric data are usually available from the school and are invaluable in interpreting later neuropsychological assessments.

Head Injury and Its Sequelae

Head injury is common and is potentially a factor in later mood and psychotic disorders as well as in cognitive impairment, epilepsy, and posttraumatic stress disorder (Chadwick 2000; Jorge

Table 1–1. Elements of the medical history and review of systems

Key elements of the medical history

- Organ systems review: heart, lung, liver, kidney, skin, joint, eye, thyroid
- Hypertension
- Diabetes
- Traumatic brain injury
- Seizures, including febrile convulsions in childhood
- Unexplained medical symptoms
- Substance misuse
- Current medication
- Family history of neuropsychiatric disorder

Key issues in the review of systems

- Constitutional symptoms: fever, malaise, weight loss, pain complaints
- Neurological symptoms: headache, blurred or double vision, impairment of balance, impairments of visual or auditory acuity, swallowing disturbance, focal or transient weakness or sensory loss, clumsiness, gait disturbance, alteration of urinary or defecatory function, altered sexual function
- Paroxysmal limbic phenomena: micropsia, macropsia, metamorphopsia, *déjà vu* and *jamais vu, déjà écouté* and *jamais écouté,* forced thoughts or emotions, depersonalization/derealization, autoscopy, paranormal experiences such as clairvoyance or telepathy
- Endocrine symptoms: heat or cold sensitivity, constipation or diarrhea, rapid heart rate, alopecia or change in texture of hair, change in skin pigmentation, change in menses
- Rheumatic disease symptoms: joint pain or swelling, mouth ulcers, dry mouth or eyes, rash, past spontaneous abortions

and Robinson 2002; McDonald et al. 2002; Sachdev et al. 2001; Seel et al. 2003). The clinician should inquire about a history of head injury in virtually every patient. The nature of the injury should be clarified by eliciting the circumstances, including risk-taking behaviors that may have predisposed to injury and the consequences for others injured in the same incident, often an emotionally powerful aspect of the event. Loss of consciousness is not a prerequisite to important sequelae; even a period of being stunned or "seeing stars" can presage later neuropsychiatric symptoms (Erlanger et al. 2003). Along with the period of loss of consciousness (coma), the clinician should establish the duration of retrograde amnesia (from last memory before the injury to the injury itself) and of posttraumatic or anterograde amnesia (from injury to recovery of the capacity for consecutive memory). The latter is often the best predictor of subsequent indices of severity of injury.

Spells

Paroxysmal disorders of neuropsychiatric interest include epilepsy, migraine, panic attacks, pseudoseizures, and episodic dyscontrol of aggression. Taking a history of an attack involves common features irrespective of the nature of the disorder. The clinician should obtain a microhistory of the events of the attack, tracking the symptoms and behavior minute by minute (or even second by second) with the patient and, if possible, an observer of the spells. The history starts with the possible presence of a prodrome, the warning of an impending attack in the hours or days before one occurs. The attack may be presaged by an aura lasting seconds to minutes. In the case of an epileptic seizure, this represents the core of the seizure itself and may carry important localizing information about the side and site of the focus. The pace and duration of the spell, from onset to peak of the ictus to termination, are important in making the differential diagnosis. For example, epileptic seizures begin abruptly; panic attacks may have a more gradual development to peak intensity. Panic attacks last much longer than seizures, the latter usually no more than a minute or two, the former often 15 minutes or more. The patient's state in the immediate postictal period is also important to the differential diagnosis; confusion and lethargy are common after an epileptic seizure but may be notably absent after a pseudoseizure. The frequency of episodes, both at present and at maximum and minimum in the past, should be established. Inquiring whether the patient has just one sort of spell or more than one is an essential prelude to establishing the frequency of spells and may also yield differential diagnostic information. Patients may have both complex partial seizures and secondarily generalized seizures, or they may have both epileptic convulsions and pseudoseizures.

By interviewing the patient and collateral informants, the clinician can usually elicit the information necessary to make a differential diagnosis. The differential diagnosis between epilepsy and pseudoseizures can be difficult, but at times, if asked properly, the patient will make the diagnosis for the clinician by reporting two kinds of seizures, one of which is clearly epileptic and the other of which is clearly dependent on emotional states. The clinician should not rely on the presence of the supposed classic features of hysteria to make this differential diagnosis, because behaviors such as pelvic thrusting and vocalization occur in epilepsy, particularly in seizures of frontal origin, which may pose particularly difficult problems in the differential diagnosis (Saygi et al. 1992).

Cognitive Symptoms

Cognitive symptoms may be overshadowed by more dramatic behavioral or mood change. Many patients will phrase their cognitive complaints in terms of memory problems, although on closer inspection the problem may lie in other domains. For example, a middle-aged nurse had experienced cardiac arrest and anoxic brain injury during a surgical procedure. Subsequently, she and her husband presented with the report that she could not remember what to do in the home. For example, they said, when she has the plan to make the beds during the day, he returns to discover she has forgotten to do so. Written reminders to carry out the activity, however, had not ameliorated her "forgetfulness"; in fact, she might spend the day sitting on the couch looking at the reminder to make the beds. This was a problem of apathy or abulia, not amnesia.

Cognitive complaints may reflect depressive ideation and depressive attentional failure (Piazzini et al. 2001). However, such complaints may also be a harbinger of dementia, albeit a weak and nonspecific predictor (Jorm et al. 2001; St John and Montgomery 2002). The clinician should establish whether forgotten material (say, an acquaintance's name or a task meant to be performed) comes to the patient later, which would suggest absent-mindedness rather than amnesia.

Complaints of a loss of capacity for divided attention or for the automatic performance of familiar tasks are highly characteristic of organic disease. A patient might report, for example, no longer being able to read and listen to the radio at the same time. Getting lost or beginning to use aids for recall, such as a notebook, are suggestive of organic cognitive failure.

Appetitive Symptoms and Personality Change

Alterations in sleep, appetite, and energy are common in idiopathic psychiatric disorders as well as transiently in the healthy population and cannot generally be interpreted as implying brain disease. Certain patterns of altered sleeping and eating behavior and personality, however, are pointers to organic disease. Excessive daytime sleepiness or sleep attacks raise the question of sleep apnea or narcolepsy—or, in a different temporal pattern, the Kleine-Levin syndrome. If possible, sleepiness (which is relieved by sleep) should be distinguished from fatigue. Snoring and morning headache, pointers to sleep apnea, may accompany excessive sleepiness and should be inquired about. Fatigue, a common symptom, generally yields little to laboratory evaluation, and thorough clinical assessment is indicated (but only limited testing) (Working Group of the Royal Australasian College of Physicians 2002). Cognitive impairment may be a consequence of sleep disruption by apnea, so this condition should be considered under the rubric of treatable factors in dementia (Naegele et al. 1998; Steiner et al. 1999).

Abnormal behavior during sleep raises the question of a parasomnia. Of particular interest is rapid eye movement behavior disorder, which may be due to a pontine lesion, but when a focal lesion is absent strongly points to ingravescent Lewy body disease (or other synucleinopathy) (Boeve et al. 2001). Abnormal nocturnal behavior associated with insomnia due to structural lesions has recently been termed *agrypnia excitata* and has been linked to lesions involving thalamic and limbic regions (Montagna and Lugaresi 2002). One such condition is fatal insomnia (familial or sporadic), a prion disease with predominant thalamic involvement. Cessation of dreaming occurs with parietal or bifrontal damage; loss of visual imagery in dreams occurs with ventral occipitotemporal damage (Solms 1995).

Patterns of abnormal eating also may have differential diagnostic value. In medial hypothalamic disease, eating behavior is marked by lack of satiety and resultant obesity. In the Klüver-Bucy syndrome of bilateral anterior temporal damage (involving the amygdala), patients mouth nonfood items. With frontal damage, patients may display altered food preferences, eating stereotypies, and the stuffing of food into the mouth, a form of utilization behavior. Increased appetite and weight gain are far more common in frontotemporal dementia than in Alzheimer's disease (Ikeda et al. 2002). A gourmand syndrome of excessive concern with fine eating has been associated with right anterior injury (Regard and Landis 1997).

Changes in sexual behavior are common consequences of brain disease. Hyposexuality is common in epilepsy, possibly as a consequence of limbic discharges, but is infrequently the subject of spontaneous complaint (Lambert 2001). A change in habitual sexual interests, quantitative or qualitative, developing in midlife suggests organic disease (Cummings 1999). Organic disease, such as the sequelae of traumatic brain injury, may be a frequent etiological factor in sexual offending and domestic violence, but the issue has been inadequately studied (DelBello et al. 1999; Rosenbaum et al. 1994). Changes in personality, such as the development of shallowness of affect, irritability, the loss of sense of humor, or a coarsening of sensibilities, may indicate ingravescent organic disease—for example, frontotemporal dementia.

Handedness

A psychiatrist who inquires about the patient's handedness has staked a fair claim to neuropsychiatric sophistication. One may accurately consider handedness (dextral, sinistral, or ambidextrous) to be a dimensional (i.e., a matter of degree) rather than a categorical trait (Annett 1998). A patient may assert right-handedness but use the left hand preferentially for certain tasks. Inquiring about a few specific tasks—writing, throwing, drawing, using scissors or a toothbrush—yields helpful information. A family history of sinistrality may also be relevant. Patients who demonstrate anomalous patterns of cognitive deficit after unilateral brain damage are of particular interest. Crossed aphasia (aphasia after right-hemisphere injury in a dextral patient) or crossed nonaphasia (absence of aphasia in a dextral patient after a left-hemisphere lesion that should cause language impairment) are well described; patterns of deficit in other localized functions are less well studied (Alexander and Annett 1996; Fischer et al. 1991).

Examining the Neuropsychiatric Patient

General Physical Examination

General Appearance

Dysmorphic features may form a pattern diagnosable as a developmental syndrome. Such syndromes may have characteristic psychiatric correlates, so-called behavioral phenotypes (Moldavsky et al. 2001). The presence of dysmorphic features in a mentally retarded patient increases the odds of finding a subtelomeric chromosomal rearrangement (Shevell et al. 2003). Psychiatric dysmorphology also includes so-called minor physical anomalies, no single one of which is pathognomonic of abnormal development. These malformations cluster in the head, hands, and feet. Examples are unusually formed or low-set ears; a double hair whorl or fine, "electric" hair; a U-shaped or broad and flat palate; and unusual patterns of creases of the hands (Trixler et al. 2001). An increased number of minor anomalies is seen in nonsyndromal mental retardation, schizophrenia, and other neurodevelopmental disorders. Some minor malformations can be assessed quantitatively, and such anthropometrics may come to play a larger role in psychiatric research (McGrath et al. 2002; Trixler et al. 2001). *Cleft lip* or *palate* is associated with brain malformations and frontal cognitive impairment (Nopoulos et al. 2002a, 2002b).

Asymmetry of the extremities (often best seen in the thumbnails) or of the cranial vault points to a developmental abnormality. The larger extremity and the smaller side of the head are ipsilateral to the abnormal cerebral hemisphere. *Short stature* is an important feature of many developmental syndromes, both common (such as fetal alcohol syndrome and Down syndrome) and uncommon (such as mitochondrial cytopathies).

Vital Signs

Fever, tachycardia, and *tachypnea* should never be ignored, even in a patient whose agitation or anxiety might seem to explain the abnormality. Abnormal vital signs are pointers to infection, dehydration, cardiac or thyroid disease, noninfectious inflammatory disease such as lupus, neuroleptic malignant syndrome, pheochromocytoma, and fatal familial insomnia—to survey some of the possibilities from the common to the rare. *Abnormal respiratory patterns* occur in hyperkinetic movement disorders (including tardive dyskinesia). *Yawning* is seen in opiate withdrawal and with serotonergic drugs (Daquin et al. 2001). *Weight loss* is an important clue to systemic disease such as neoplasia; it should not be dismissed without further consideration even in a patient with depression, which may—but may not—account for the weight loss. *Weight gain* similarly may point to limbic or systemic disease, especially an endocrinopathy (for example, the centripetal obesity and buffalo hump of Cushing's syndrome), or may reflect toxicity of psychotropic drugs.

Skin

Alopecia is a feature of lupus, hypothyroidism, and reactions to psychiatric and other medicines. *Hirsutism* may betoken various endocrinopathies, including congenital adrenal hyperplasia, which may have interesting neuropsychiatric correlates (Herzog et al. 2001; Jacobs et al. 1999). The *neurocutaneous syndromes* have characteristic manifestations: adenoma sebaceum (facial angiofibromas), ash-leaf macules, depigmented nevi, and shagreen patches (thickened, yellowish skin over the lumbosacral area) in tuberous sclerosis; a port-wine stain (typically involving both upper and lower eyelids) in Sturge-Weber syndrome; neurofibromas, café au lait spots, and axillary freckling in neurofibromatosis.

Skin disorders are particularly useful signs of the rheumatic disorders (Ovsiew and Utset 2002). A pink periungual rash, a slightly raised and tender erythematous rash involving both cheeks but sparing the nasolabial folds (malar rash), and a hyperkeratotic and hypopigmented scarring eruption (discoid lupus) are features of lupus erythematosus. A netlike violaceous rash involving the trunk and lower extremities (livedo reticularis) is associated with Sneddon's syndrome of cerebrovascular disease and dementia and with the presence of antiphospholipid antibodies. Palpable *purpura* is indicative of vasculitis.

Head

Head circumference should be measured in patients with a question of developmental disorder. Although height and weight need to be taken into account along with gender, roughly the normal range for adult men is 54–60 cm (21.25–23.5 inches); for women, 52–58 cm (20.5–22.75 inches) (Bushby et al. 1992). *Old skull fracture* or *intracranial surgery* usually leaves palpable evidence.

Eyes

Exophthalmos usually indicates Graves' disease. A space-occupying lesion should be considered especially if the exophthalmos is unilateral. The *Kayser-Fleischer ring* is a brownish-green discoloration at the limbus of the cornea; it sensitively and specifically—although imperfectly (Demirkiran et al. 1996)—indicates neuropsychiatric Wilson's disease (but is much less sensitive in hepatic presentations of the disease). *Dry eyes,* along with dry mouth, raise the question of Sjögren's syndrome, although drug toxicity and the aging process are common confounds. Inflammation in the anterior portion of the eye, *uveitis,* is manifested by pain, redness, and a constricted pupil; this is commonly associated with connective tissue disease. In general, ophthalmological consultation can be useful in a puzzling case involving potential rheumatological disease (Hamideh and Prete 2001). The pupils, optic disks, visual fields, and eye movements are discussed later under "Neurological Examination."

Mouth

Oral ulcers can be seen in lupus, Behçet's disease, and other connective tissue disease. *Dry mouth* is a part of the sicca syndrome. Vitamin B_{12} deficiency produces *atrophic glossitis,* a smooth, painful, red tongue.

Heart and Vessels

A *carotid bruit* indicates turbulent flow in the vessel but is a poor predictor of the degree or potential risk of the vascular lesion (Shorr et al. 1998). A thickened, tender *temporal artery* points to giant-cell arteritis; here the physical examination is an excellent guide to clinical significance (Salvarani et al. 2002). Cardiac valvular disease, marked by cardiac *murmurs,* is important in assessing the cause of stroke, and congestive failure or infection may be relevant in delirium. In a schizophrenic patient, a murmur may raise the question of the velo-cardio-facial syndrome. Patients with developmental disabilities may have multiple anomalies, including structural heart disease.

Neck

A *short, thick neck* may predispose to obstructive sleep apnea. *Palpation of the thyroid* should help in the diagnosis of hyperthyroidism and hypothyroidism.

Extremities

Joint inflammation as a pointer to systemic rheumatic disease is distinguished from noninflammatory degenerative joint disease (osteoarthritis) by the presence of swelling, warmth, and erythema and is characteristically seen in wrists, ankles, and metacarpophalangeal joints, as opposed to the involvement of the base of the thumb, distal interphalangeal joints, and spine seen in degenerative joint disease. *Raynaud's phenomenon* and *sclerodactyly* are signs of connective tissue disease. The *warm, dry hands* of hyperthyroidism are a differentiating feature from idiopathic anxiety disorders, in which the hands are cool and clammy.

Neurological Examination

Olfaction

Hyposmia is common in neurological disease, but local disease of the nasal mucosa must be excluded before a defect is taken to be of neuropsychiatric significance. Assessment of olfaction is often ignored ("cranial nerves II through XII normal"), but it is easily performed and gives clues to the integrity of regions that are otherwise hard to assess, notably the orbitofrontal cortex. (The olfactory nerve lies underneath the orbitofrontal cortex; projections go to the olfactory tubercle, the entorhinal and piriform cortex in the temporal lobes, the amygdala, and the orbitofrontal cortex.) Testing of olfaction is best performed using a floral odorant (Pinching 1977) such as scented lip balms, which are inexpensive and simple to carry. Although a distinction can be made between the threshold for odor detection and that for identification of the stimulus, with differing anatomies, at the bedside without special equipment the best one can achieve is recognition of a decrement in sensitivity (i.e., whether the patient smells anything, even without being able to identify it).

Eyes

Impairment of *visual acuity* is a sign of neural dysfunction only after refractive error—that is, ocular disease—is corrected. In the absence of the patient's corrective lenses, a pinhole can be used at the bedside. *Pupillary* dilation may indicate anticholinergic toxicity; pupillary constriction is a characteristic feature of opiate toxicity. Argyll Robertson pupils are bilateral, small, irregular, and reactive to accommodation but not to light; the finding is characteristic of paretic neurosyphilis but is also present in other conditions (Dacso and Bortz 1989). *Papilledema* indicates increased intracranial pressure; the earliest and most sensitive feature, before hyperemia or blurring of the disk margins, is loss of venous pulsations at the optic disk (Jacks and Miller 2003). However, the finding is nonspecific; that is, the presence of spontaneous venous pulsations reliably indicates normal intracranial pressure, but its absence does not mean that pressure is elevated. A homonymous upper-quadrant *field defect* is present when temporal lobe disease affects Meyer's loop, the portion of the optic radiation that dips into the temporal lobe (Tecoma et al. 1993). A field defect in a delirious patient may point to stroke as the cause of delirium (Caplan et al. 1986; Devinsky et al. 1988). The normal spontaneous *blink rate* is 16±8/minute. Reduced central dopamine function, as in parkinsonism, is associated with a reduction in blink rate. An increased blink rate or paroxysms of blinking are sometimes seen in acutely psychotic patients. Impairment of voluntary eye opening may be present in association with extrapyramidal signs, for example in progressive supranuclear palsy (Lamberti et al. 2002). Reflex eye opening and voluntary eye closure are normal, and sensory tricks may assist in eye opening (Defazio et al. 1998). In blepharospasm, as opposed to an impairment of voluntary eye opening, the brows are lowered below the superior margin of the orbits (Grandas and Esteban 1994). Impairment of voluntary eye closure may be seen after damage to the frontal or basal ganglia (Ghika et al. 1988; Russell 1980).

Both saccadic and pursuit *eye movements* should be examined. The former are assessed by asking the patient to look without a target to the left and the right, up and down, and at the examiner's finger on the left, right, up, and down. Pursuit eye movements are examined by asking the patient to follow the examiner's moving finger in both the horizontal and vertical planes. These maneuvers test supranuclear control of eye movements; the oculocephalic maneuver (doll's-head eyes) (i.e., moving the patient's head) tests the brainstem pathways and may be added to the examination if saccades or pursuit is abnormal. Limitation of voluntary upgaze is common in the healthy elderly. Limitation of voluntary downgaze, however, in a patient with extrapyramidal signs or frontal cognitive impairment suggests progressive supranuclear palsy. Slowed saccades are characteristic of Huntington's disease. Impairment of initiation of voluntary saccades (saccade initiation failure), requiring a head thrust or head turning, amounts to an apraxia of gaze and is seen in developmental disorders as well as Huntington's disease, Gaucher's disease type III, and parietal damage (Harris et al. 1998, 1999; Leigh et al. 1983). Together with impairment of reaching under visual guidance and simultanagnosia, apraxia of gaze (also called psychic paralysis of gaze or ocular apraxia) forms the Balint syndrome. Impairment of inhibition of saccades represents a visual grasp, with forced gaze at environmental stimuli, and is associated with prefrontal dysfunction (Everling and Fischer 1998; Ghika et al. 1995). This can be sought by placing stimuli (a finger and a fist) in the left and right visual fields of the patient and asking the patient to look at the fist when the finger moves, and vice versa. The test forms a useful part of a screening battery for encephalopathy in acquired immunodeficiency syndrome and probably in other conditions (Power et al. 1995).

Facial Movement

Both spontaneous movements of emotional expression and movement to command should be tested. After lesions involving pyramidal pathways, spontaneous movements may be relatively spared when the face is hemiparetic for voluntary movements. Contrariwise, in nonpyramidal motor disorders, voluntary movement may be possible despite a lateralized defect of spontaneous movement (Hopf et al. 1992). Lesions causing emotional facial paresis may involve the supplementary motor area, basal ganglia, internal capsule, thalamus, or medial temporal lobe. The last is of particular interest because a unilateral paresis of emotional facial movement is of lateralizing significance in temporal lobe epilepsy (Jacob et al. 2003). The most severe form of the pyramidal disorder with sparing of spontaneous movement is seen after bilateral anterior opercular lesions, the Foix-Chavany-Marie syndrome (Broussolle et al. 1996; Szabo et al. 2002).

Speech

The *mute* patient, despite alertness, makes no attempt at spoken communication. The examiner should assess nonspeech movements of the relevant musculature, for example, tongue movements, swallowing, and coughing. Other means of communication should be attempted, such as gesture, writing, or pointing on a letter-board or word-board. Mutism may occur at the onset of aphemia or transcortical aphasia due to vascular lesions or late in the course of frontotemporal dementia or primary progressive aphasia.

Patterns of *dysarthria* are distinctive but are hard to convey in print. In pyramidal dysarthria speech is slowed, strained, and slurred; in ataxic dysarthria speech is slowed with imprecise articulation and equalization of or erratic stressing of syllables (scanning speech); in extrapyramidal dysarthria speech is hypophonic and monotonous, tailing off with longer utterances; and in bulbar dysarthria speech is nasal, breathy, and slurred. *Apraxia of speech* refers to inconsistent and slowed articulation, limited variation of volume, and abnormal prosody, seen characteristically with lesions of the left insula (Dronkers 1996). Occasional patients with dysarthria due to lesions in motor or premotor cortices or their subjacent white matter in the language-dominant hemisphere will show a language pattern interpreted by listeners as a foreign accent (Kurowski et al. 1996). *Echolalia* refers to automatic repetition of the interlocutor's speech or of words heard in the environment; sometimes pronouns are reversed, grammar corrected, or well-known phrases completed. *Palilalia* is the automatic repetition of the patient's own final words or phrase, with increasing rapidity and decreasing volume; it is an extrapyramidal sign. *Stuttering* is the repetition, prolongation, and arrest of sounds. Usually a developmental syndrome, it may also emerge as a result of acquired brain disease, in which case the dystonic facial movements characteristic of the developmental form are not seen (Ciabarra et al. 2000). Acquired stuttering is associated with extrapyramidal disease and strokes, but developmental stuttering that had been overcome may also reappear with the onset of parkinsonism or after stroke (Shahed and Jankovic 2001).

Abnormalities of Movement

Weakness due to muscle disease, peripheral nerve disease, or lower motor neuron disease is associated with atrophy, fasciculations, characteristic distributions, loss of reflexes, and (in the case of muscle disease) muscle tenderness. These disorders are reviewed in textbooks of neurology (e.g., Duus 1998). Of greater relevance to the examiner seeking evidence of cerebral dysfunction is pyramidal weakness. This is greatest in the distal musculature and is marked by reduced control of fine movements. The deficit in fine motor control can be elicited by asking the patient to touch each finger to the thumb of the same hand, quickly and repeatedly. Pyramidal weakness is accompanied by increased muscle tone in a spastic pattern (flexors in the upper extremity, extensors in the lower extremity, with the sudden loss of increased tone during passive movement, the clasp-knife phenomenon), brisk tendon jerks, and the presence of abnormal reflexes such as Babinski's sign (discussed later). A nonpyramidal form of central motor dysfunction is seen with lesions of the caudate nucleus or premotor cortex. These patients show clumsiness, decreased spontaneous use of affected limbs, and apparent weakness but production of full strength with coaxing. Pronation of the outstretched supinated arms may disclose a subtle pyramidal deficit; similarly, the forearm rolling test is performed by asking the patient to roll the forearms around each other first in one direction and then in the other, looking for one side that moves less, thus appearing to be an axis with the other circling around.

Apart from spasticity, increased *muscle tone* can also have the pattern of paratonic rigidity, or *Gegenhalten*. This is manifested by an erratic, pseudoactive increase in resistance to passive movement. The fluctuating quality of the resistance reflects the presence of both oppositional and facilitory aspects of the patient's response. The facilitory aspect can be evoked by repeatedly flexing and extending the patient's arm at the elbow, then abruptly ceasing and letting go when the arm is extended; the abnormal response, facilitory paratonia, is for the patient to continue the sequence by flexion (Beversdorf and Heilman 1998). Hypertonus due to extrapyramidal disease has the features of increased tone in both extensors and flexors and throughout the range of movement, so-called lead-pipe rigidity. The cogwheel or ratchety feel to the rigidity is imparted by a coexisting tremor and is not intrinsic to the hypertonus; when paratonic rigidity co-occurs with a metabolic tremor, a delirious patient may mistakenly be thought to have Parkinson's disease.

Gait should always be tested, if only by focused attention to the patient's entering or leaving the room. Attention should be paid to the patient's station, postural reflexes, stride length and base, and turning (Nutt et al. 1993). *Postural reflexes* can be assessed by asking the patient to stand in a comfortable fashion, then pushing gently on the chest or back, with care taken to avoid a fall. Gait should be stressed by asking the patient to walk in tandem fashion and on the outer aspects of the feet. Inability to perform tandem gait reveals mild ataxia, often referable to cerebellar vermis dysfunction; posturing of the upper extremities during stressed gait reflects nonpyramidal motor dysfunction. A common diagnostic problem is to differentiate idiopathic parkinsonism from parkinsonism due to subcortical vascular disease. The latter shows disturbance of gait disproportionate to other leg movements, the occasional presence of a wide base, an upright posture, preservation of arm swing, absence of festination, relative sparing of upper body movement, absence of rest tremor, and poor response to levodopa (FitzGerald and Jankovic 1989; Nutt et al. 1993; Thompson and Marsden 1987; Yamanouchi and Nagura 1997). Similar findings are present in hydrocephalus.

Akinesia is manifested by delay in initiation, slowness of execution, and difficulty with complex or simultaneous movements. Mild akinesia may be observed in the patient's lack of spontaneous movements of the body while sitting or of the face, or elicited by asking the patient to make repeated large-amplitude taps of the forefinger on the thumb (looking for decay of the amplitude). Akinesia is characteristically accompanied by rigidity, but pure akinesia is occasionally seen. These plus rest tremor and postural instability represent the core features of the parkinsonian syndrome, seen not only in idiopathic Parkinson's disease but in several other degenerative, Parkinson-plus disorders such as progressive supranuclear palsy and multiple system atrophy as well as in vascular white matter disease. Rest tremor is less common in these other disorders than in idiopathic Parkinson's disease.

Dystonia is sustained muscle contraction with consequent twisting movements or abnormal postures. Typically dystonia in the upper extremity is manifested as hyperpronation; in the lower extremity, as inversion of the foot with plantar flexion. Dystonia may occur only with certain actions, such as writer's cramp; focally or segmentally, such as blepharospasm or oculogyric crisis; or in a generalized pattern, such as torsion dystonia associated with mutations in the *DYT1* gene. The symptoms and signs often violate a common-sense idea of how things ought to be in organic disease; the risk is of attributing to psychogenesis an organic phenomenon that is not known to the clinician. For example, a patient with early torsion dystonia may be able to run but not walk, because the latter action elicits leg dystonia, or a patient with intense neck muscle contraction may be able to bring the head to the midline by a light touch on the chin. Such a *geste antagoniste* or sensory trick is diagnostic of dystonia.

Tremor is a regular oscillating movement around a joint. In *rest tremor,* the movement occurs in a relaxed, supported extremity and is reduced by action. Often an upper-extremity rest tremor is amplified by ambulation. The tremor frequency is usually 4–8 Hz. This is the distinctive tremor of Parkinson's disease. In *postural tremor,* sustained posture, such as holding the arms outstretched, elicits tremor. Hereditary essential tremor presents as postural tremor, predominantly in upper extremities but also at times involving the head, jaw, and voice. A coarse, irregular, rapid postural tremor is often seen in metabolic encephalopathy. In *intention tremor,* the active limb oscillates more prominently when approaching its target, such as touching with the index finger the examiner's finger. Maximizing the range of the movement increases the sensitivity of the test. Intention tremor is one form of *kinetic tremor,* that is, tremor elicited by movement; another sort is tremor elicited by a specific action, such as writing tremor or orthostatic tremor on standing upright. To characterize tremor, the examiner observes the patient with arms supported and fully at rest, then with arms outstretched and pronated, then with arms abducted to 90° at the shoulders and bent at the elbows while the hands are held palms down with the fingers pointing at each other in front of the chest. The patient should also be observed during ambulation. Anxiety exaggerates tremor; this normal phenomenon—for example, when the patient is conscious of being observed—should not be mistaken for psychogenesis. A good test for psychogenic tremor relies on the fact that although organic tremor may vary in amplitude, it varies little in frequency. A patient can be asked to tap a hand at a frequency different from the tremor frequency; if another tremulous body part entrains to the tapped frequency, psychogenic tremor is likely. The *coactivation sign* of psychogenic tremor refers to the breakdown of increased tone and tremor during passive movement of the affected extremity (Deuschl et al. 1998).

Choreic movements are random and arrhythmic movements of small amplitude that dance over the patient's body. They may be more evident when the patient is engaged in an activity such as ambulation. When the movements are of large amplitude and forceful, the disorder is called *ballism.* Ballistic movements are usually unilateral.

Myoclonus is a sudden, jerky, shocklike movement. It is more discontinuous than chorea or tremor. The negative of myoclonus is *asterixis,* a sudden lapse of muscle contraction in the context of attempted maintenance of posture. Both phenomena, but more sensitively asterixis, are common in toxic-metabolic encephalopathy (not just hepatic encephalopathy). Asterixis should be sought by observation of the patient's attempt to maintain extension of the hands with the arms outstretched; it is pathognomonic for organic disease and is never seen in acute idiopathic psychosis or other nonorganic disorders. Myoclonus occurs in many other settings and is an important diagnostic pointer for nonconvulsive generalized status epilepticus, Hashimoto's encephalopathy, and Creutzfeldt-Jakob disease. Unilateral asterixis may rarely be seen in parietal, frontal, or (most often) thalamic structural disease (Rio et al. 1995; Tatu et al. 2000).

Tics are sudden, jerky movements as well, but they may be more complex than myoclonic jerks and are subjectively characterized by an impulse to perform the act and a sense of relief for having done so (or mounting tension otherwise). Compulsions are not easy to differentiate from complex tics; the tiqueur may, like the patient with compulsions, report deliberately performing the act. Repetitive behavior superficially like compulsions may occur in organic disease but represents environment-driven behavior rather than having the same subjective structure as compulsive behavior. For example, a patient with frontal disease may repeatedly touch an alluring object without an elicitable subjective impulse and without anxiety if separated from the object. However, organic obsessions and compulsions occur as well and have been associated with cortical and basal ganglia lesions (Berthier et al. 1996). These do not differ phenomenologically from obsessions and compulsions in the idiopathic disorder, but the patients have later age at onset and lack a pertinent family history.

Akathisia is defined by both its subjective and its objective features. The patient expresses an urge to move and exhibits motor restlessness—for example, by shifting weight from foot to foot while standing (marching in place). Often psychotic or cognitively impaired patients cannot convey the subjective experience clearly, and the examiner must be alert for the objective signs in order to differentiate akathisia from agitation due to anxiety or psychosis. The complaints and the signs in akathisia are referable to the lower extremities: the anxious patient may wring his or her hands, the akathisic patient shuffles his or her feet. Watching the patient stand is an essential part of the examination. Myoclonic jerks of the legs may be evident in the recumbent patient. The phenomenon occurs in idiopathic Parkinson's disease and with drug-induced dopamine blockade, but also rarely with extensive frontal or temporal structural lesions (Sachdev and Kruk 1996).

Ataxia is a disorder of coordinating the rate, range, and force of movement and is characteristic of damage to the cerebellum and its connections. With the limbs, the patient overshoots or undershoots the target (dysmetria), because of impaired determination of movement distance. Oscillation of the reaching limb amounts to intention tremor. Asking the patient to touch the examiner's finger, then his or her own nose, tests this system. Accurately touching one's own nose with eyes closed requires both cerebellar and proprioceptive function. Eye movements also may be hypermetric or hypometric. Difficulty in performing rapid alternating movements, such as supination and pronation of the hand or tapping of the foot, is called *dysdiadochokinesia.* The failure of coordination of movement is also demonstrated by loss of check, which should not be elicited by arranging for the patient to hit himself or herself when the examiner's hand is removed. In the normal situation, if the outstretched arms are tapped, only a slight waver is produced; the ataxic patient fails to damp the movement. Gait may be affected by midline cerebellar (vermis) disease in the absence of limb ataxia, which is related to cerebellar hemisphere disease. Gait is unsteady, with irregular stride length and a widened base. (In the nonataxic subject, the feet nearly touch at their nearest point; even a few inches of separation represents widening of the base.) Gait and limb ataxia may be complemented by ataxic dysarthria and by eye movement disorders, including nystagmus (usually gaze-paretic), slowed saccades, saccadic pursuit, and gaze apraxia.

The core of the *catatonic* syndrome is a mute, motionless state; variably added are abnormal movements, including grimacing, stereotypy, echopraxia, and catalepsy. The latter, known also as *flexibilitas cerea* (waxy flexibility), refers to posturing of a limb in the position in which it is placed by the examiner, or in some other unnatural position. It is infrequent in catatonia, and it can be seen apart from the catatonic syndrome in patients with contralateral parietal lesions (the levitation of the parietal arm [Ghika et al. 1998; Saver et al. 1993]). *Catatonic excitement* refers to the sudden eruption into overactivity of a motionless catatonic patient. Such a development probably reveals psychotic mania. The catatonic syndrome occurs in the course of schizophrenia or mood disorder, or without other psychopathology as idiopathic catatonia, or in the setting of acute cerebral metabolic or structural derangements (Barnes et al. 1986). In the latter case it is best thought of as a nonspecific reaction pattern, such as is delirium, requiring a comprehensive clinical and laboratory evaluation to seek the cause of the behavioral disturbance. An important instance is catatonia as part of the neuroleptic malignant syndrome, the diagnosis of which requires exclusion of other causes of encephalopathy, notably systemic infection. Catatonia is thus a medical emergency, requiring prompt attention to diagnostic evaluation as well as supportive care (fluids, nutrition, and measures to avoid complications of immobility, including venous thrombosis).

Abnormalities of Sensation

Disorders of sensation may be difficult to assess reliably in patients with cognitive and behavior disorders. Nonetheless, several points should be familiar to the neuropsychiatrist. Distal loss of sensation, often accompanied by loss of ankle jerks, is characteristic of peripheral neuropathy. Often all modalities of sensation are disturbed. If proprioception is sufficiently reduced, Romberg's sign will be present. Romberg's sign means that closing the eyes produces a substantial increase in impairment of balance; it is elicited by asking the patient to stand, allowing the patient to seek a comfortably balanced position, then asking the patient to close the eyes (while ensuring against a fall). This is a sign of sensory impairment, originally described in the context of dorsal root damage from the tabes dorsalis, although it only imperfectly excludes a cerebellar contribution to imbalance (Lanska and Goetz 2000).

Loss of sensation from sensory cortex injury is classically limited to complex discriminations, such as graphesthesia (recognizing numbers written on the palm), stereognosis (identifying unseen objects in the hand), and two-point discrimination (telling whether the examiner is touching with one or two points, as these come closer together in space). These findings should be sought if features of the history or examination point to abnormalities in the parietal cortex. Patients with parietal stroke may also have a pseudothalamic sensory syndrome, with impairments in elementary sensory modalities and subsequent dysesthesia, or other anomalous patterns of sensory loss (Bassetti et al. 1993). At times these patients present with pseudomotor deficits: ataxia, fluctuating muscle tone and strength (dependent in part on visual cueing), or levitation and awkward positioning of the arm contralateral (or at times ipsilateral) to the lesion (Ghika et al. 1998). In the acute phase, the combination of deficits can amount to motor helplessness as a result of the loss of sensory input to regions in which motor programs arise.

Soft Signs

Batteries of soft signs include assessments of sensorimotor integration and motor control. From the corpus of test batteries (Sanders and Keshavan 1998), a few simple maneuvers can be extracted that may make a contribution to the neurological examination of the patient with a mental presentation. While the patient is touching each finger to the thumb, as described earlier under "Abnormalities of Movement," the examiner can watch the opposite hand for mirror movements. Obligatory bimanual synkinesias are seen specifically in disorders of the pyramidal pathways, such as the Klippel-Feil syndrome, and in agenesis of the corpus callosum, but also in putative neurodevelopmental disorders such as schizophrenia (Rasmussen 1993). Asking the patient, with eyes closed, to report whether the examiner is touching one or the other hand (with the patient's hands on the patient's lap), or one or the other side of the face, or a combination, makes up the face-hand test. The examiner touches the left hand and right face simultaneously. If the patient reports only the touch on the face (i.e., extinguishes the peripheral stimulus), then the examiner can prompt (once), "Anywhere else?" Then the examiner touches the right hand and left cheek, left hand and left cheek, right hand and right cheek, both hands, and both cheeks. Extinction of the peripheral stimulus is the pathological response and has been associated with schizophrenia and dementia (Sanders and Keshavan 2002). Motor sequencing tasks include the alternating fists (Oseretsky) test: with arms extended and palms face down, the patient is asked to make one hand into a fist, then the other, so that one hand is open, the other clenched, alternatingly. An abnormal response has both hands open or closed at the same time. The ring/fist or fist/edge/palm tests, devised by Luria (1966), require the patient to perform a sequence of movements without perseveration.

Abnormal Reflexes

Babinski's sign is the hallmark of the neurological examination (van Gijn 1996). It should be elicited by stroking the lateral aspect of the foot from back to front, with the leg extended at the knee, using a pointed object such as an orange stick or a key. The response of extension of the great toe with or without fanning of the other toes indicates corticospinal tract disease. The pathological response represents disinhibition of a flexor synergy that over the course of early development has come under pyramidal inhibition. Two confounding factors in assessment of Babinski's sign are the striatal toe and the plantar grasp. The striatal toe is extension of the hallux without fanning of the other toes or a flexion synergy in the other muscles of flexion of the leg (Winkler et al. 2002). It may occur in patients with Parkinson's disease in the absence of evidence of pyramidal dysfunction. The toe grasp, the lower-extremity equivalent of the more familiar palmar grasp, may mask an extensor response to lateral foot stimulation when stimulation on the plantar surface brings about flexion of the toes. Hoffmann's sign—flexion of the thumb elicited by snapping of the distal phalanx of the patient's middle finger—is an upper-extremity sign of pyramidal dysfunction, although it is sometimes present bilaterally in subjects with normal pyramidal function. Loss of abdominal reflexes, ascertained by stroking the abdomen from medial to lateral in the four quadrants, also reflects pyramidal dysfunction.

A group of reflexes are thought to represent the emergence of "primitive" motor patterns due to cerebral disease. These are not different conceptually from Babinski's sign, which also reflects disinhibition of a primitive motor synergy as discussed above, but do not point specifically to corticospinal pathways. Moreover, they are far less specific for the presence of brain disease, often being present in subjects without brain disease (Schott and Rossor 2003). For this reason, their presence must be interpreted with care. These primitive reflexes include the following:

- The grasp reflex is flexion of the fingers and adduction of the thumb with stroking of the patient's palm during distraction and despite instructions to relax. It is associated with disease of the contralateral supplementary motor area (Hashimoto and Tanaka 1998). The toe grasp (mentioned earlier), seldom present in the absence of palmar grasp, also points to medial frontal disease. The groping reflex, also called the instinctive grasp reflex, involves active movements of the hand and extremity to pursue the visual or tactile stimulus. This sign is associated with damage to the contralateral cingulate gyrus (Hashimoto and Tanaka 1998).
- Avoidance—extension of the wrist and fingers in response to the same stimulus as the grasp—is a less well-known sign that points to contralateral parietal cortex abnormality (Vilensky and Gilman 1997). A more extreme manifestation of parietal damage has been called rejection behavior (Mori and Yamadori 1989).

- The snout reflex is displayed by puckering of the lips in response to tapping on the philtrum (between the nose and the upper lip). Sucking and rooting reflexes—in which sucking is elicited by a stimulus on or in the mouth and the stimulus is sought out by turning the mouth—are likewise primitive reflexes (Schott and Rossor 2003). These are to be distinguished from the pouting reflex, elicited by tapping on the lips (often on a tongue blade placed over the lips), which is merely hyperreflexia in the affected region, akin to an exaggerated jaw jerk.
- Myerson's sign is elicited by regular (1/second) taps on the glabella (with the tapping hand outside the patient's visual field) and is present in parkinsonism and in diffuse brain disease. Ordinarily, such tapping produces a few blinks; a failure to habituate, indicated by continued blinking with continued tapping, is the abnormal phenomenon.

Conclusion

> "You see, but you do not observe [said Holmes to Watson]. The distinction is clear. For example, you have frequently seen the steps which lead up from the hall to this room."
> "Frequently."
> "How often?"
> "Well, some hundreds of times."
> "Then how many are there?"
> "How many? I don't know."
> "Quite so! You have not observed. And yet you have seen."
>
> *From "A Scandal in Bohemia"*
> *(Doyle and Baring-Gould 1967)*

Making observations requires focused looking, based on hypothesis and on expectation that arises from knowledge and theory. When told that a patient has a "wide-based gait," I often ask the student or resident how far apart (how widely spaced laterally) the feet are during normal gait. Certainly if seeing were observing, everyone would know the answer to the question. As I indicated in the introduction to this chapter, it is not possible to perform an examination that is "complete" "from head to foot"; to the contrary, performing all elements of the physical examination without hypotheses in mind would likely result in a chaotic welter of impressions. Based on knowledge of neuropsychiatric differential diagnosis, the clinician can conduct a useful examination that is brief without being cursory. For example, as a screening neurological examination, after examining saccadic and pursuit eye movements and perhaps inhibition of reflexive saccades, the examiner can observe the patient's outstretched, pronated arms; ask the patient to extend the hands at the wrists; tap the arms one by one from above; ask the patient to make fists alternately with the two hands; then supinate the arms and ask the patient to close his or her eyes; then after a few seconds ask the patient to touch his or her nose with each index finger alternately with the eyes still closed. All of the following have then been assessed in a matter of a minute or two: postural and intention tremor, asterixis and myoclonus, loss of check, motor sequencing, a pronator sign, and dysmetria. Doing this in addition to testing muscle tone (including a test for facilitory paratonia), observing the patient's natural and stressed gait, checking tendon jerks and abnormal reflexes, and examining sensation within the patient's ability to cooperate (at least with Romberg's maneuver) takes just a few minutes. Although it does not elucidate disorders of muscle, nerve, and spinal cord, this brief examination provides a rather extensive assessment of the central sensorimotor organization.

With experience, the neuropsychiatric examiner can construct a method of surveying the organ systems by history and examination and performing a more detailed examination of the elementary functions of the brain. The elements of the examination will depend on the clinical situation; some elements will be present in all examinations, others will be chosen for the purpose at hand from the examiner's tool kit. Such an examination should be within the capacity of any psychiatrist providing diagnostic evaluations.

References

Alexander MP, Annett M: Crossed aphasia and related anomalies of cerebral organization: case reports and a genetic hypothesis. Brain Lang 55:213–239, 1996

Andreasen NC, Black DW: Introductory Textbook of Psychiatry, 3rd Edition. Washington, DC, American Psychiatric Publishing, 2001

Annett M: Handedness and cerebral dominance: the right shift theory. J Neuropsychiatry Clin Neurosci 10:459–469, 1998

Barnes MP, Saunders M, Walls TJ, et al: The syndrome of Karl Ludwig Kahlbaum. J Neurol Neurosurg Psychiatry 49:991–996, 1986

Bassetti C, Bogousslavsky J, Regli F: Sensory syndromes in parietal stroke. Neurology 43:1942–1949, 1993

Berthier ML, Kulisevsky J, Gironell A, et al: Obsessive-compulsive disorder associated with brain lesions: clinical phenomenology, cognitive function, and anatomic correlates. Neurology 47:353–361, 1996

Beversdorf DQ, Heilman KM: Facilitory paratonia and frontal lobe functioning. Neurology 51:968–971, 1998

Boeve BF, Silber MH, Ferman TJ, et al: Association of REM sleep behavior disorder and neurodegenerative disease may reflect an underlying synucleinopathy. Mov Disord 16:622–630, 2001

Brodal A: Self-observations and neuro-anatomical considerations after a stroke. Brain 96:675–694, 1973

Broussolle E, Bakchine S, Tommasi M, et al: Slowly progressive anarthria with late anterior opercular syndrome: a variant form of frontal cortical atrophy syndromes. J Neurol Sci 144:44–58, 1996

Bushby KMD, Cole T, Matthews JNS, et al: Centiles for adult head circumference. Arch Dis Child 67:1286–1287, 1992

Caplan LR, Kelly M, Kase CS, et al: Infarcts of the inferior division of the right middle cerebral artery: mirror image of Wernicke's aphasia. Neurology 36:1015–1020, 1986

Chadwick D: Seizures and epilepsy after traumatic brain injury. Lancet 355:334–336, 2000

Chapman LF, Wolff HG: Disease of the neopallium and impairment of the highest integrative functions. Med Clin North Am 42:677–689, 1958

Chapman LF, Thetford WN, Berlin L, et al: Highest integrative functions in man during stress, in Brain and Human Behavior. Edited by Solomon HC, Cobb S, Penfield W. Baltimore, MD, Williams & Wilkins, 1958, pp 491–534

Ciabarra AM, Elkind MS, Roberts JK, et al: Subcortical infarction resulting in acquired stuttering. J Neurol Neurosurg Psychiatry 69:546–549, 2000

Cummings JL: Neuropsychiatry of sexual deviations, in Neuropsychiatry and Mental Health Services. Edited by Ovsiew F. Washington, DC, American Psychiatric Press, 1999, pp 363–384

Dacso CC, Bortz DL: Significance of the Argyll Robertson pupil in clinical medicine. Am J Med 86:199–202, 1989

Daquin G, Micallef J, Blin O: Yawning. Sleep Med Rev 5:299–312, 2001

Defazio G, Livrea P, Lamberti P, et al: Isolated so-called apraxia of eyelid opening: report of 10 cases and a review of the literature. Eur Neurol 39:204–210, 1998

DelBello MP, Soutullo CA, Zimmerman ME, et al: Traumatic brain injury in individuals convicted of sexual offenses with and without bipolar disorder. Psychiatry Res 89:281–286, 1999

Demirkiran M, Jankovic J, Lewis RA, et al: Neurologic presentation of Wilson disease without Kayser-Fleischer rings. Neurology 46:1040–1043, 1996

Deuschl G, Koster B, Lucking CH, et al: Diagnostic and pathophysiological aspects of psychogenic tremors. Mov Disord 13:294–302, 1998

Devinsky O, Bear D, Volpe BT: Confusional states following posterior cerebral artery infarction. Arch Neurol 45:160–163, 1988

Dolan RJ: Emotion, cognition, and behavior. Science 298:1191–1194, 2002

Doyle AC, Baring-Gould WS: The Annotated Sherlock Holmes; the Four Novels and the Fifty-Six Short Stories Complete. New York, CN Potter, 1967

Dronkers NF: A new brain region for coordinating speech articulation. Nature 384:159–161, 1996

Duus P: Topical Diagnosis in Neurology, 3rd Edition. New York, Thieme, 1998

Erlanger D, Kaushik T, Cantu R, et al: Symptom-based assessment of the severity of a concussion. J Neurosurg 98:477–484, 2003

Everling S, Fischer B: The antisaccade: a review of basic research and clinical studies. Neuropsychologia 36:885–899, 1998

Fischer RS, Alexander MP, Gabriel C, et al: Reversed lateralization of cognitive functions in right handers. Exceptions to classical aphasiology. Brain 114 (pt 1A):245–261, 1991

FitzGerald PM, Jankovic J: Lower body parkinsonism: evidence for vascular etiology. Mov Disord 4:249–260, 1989

Ghika J, Regli F, Assal G, et al: Impossibilité à la fermeture volontaire des paupières: discussion sur les troubles supranucléaires de la fermeture palpébrale à partir de 2 cas, avec revue de la littérature. Schweiz Arch Neurol Psychiatr 139(6):5–21, 1988

Ghika J, Tennis M, Growdon J, et al: Environment-driven responses in progressive supranuclear palsy. J Neurol Sci 130:104–111, 1995

Ghika J, Ghika-Schmid F, Bogousslavsky J: Parietal motor syndrome: a clinical description in 32 patients in the acute phase of pure parietal strokes studied prospectively. Clin Neurol Neurosurg 100:271–282, 1998

Ghika-Schmid F, van Melle G, Guex P, et al: Subjective experience and behavior in acute stroke: the Lausanne Emotion in Acute Stroke Study. Neurology 52:22–28, 1999

Goldstein K: The Organism: A Holistic Approach to Biology Derived From Pathological Data in Man (1934). New York, Zone Books, 1995

Grandas F, Esteban A: Eyelid motor abnormalities in progressive supranuclear palsy. J Neural Transm 42 (suppl):33–41, 1994

Hamideh F, Prete PE: Ophthalmologic manifestations of rheumatic diseases. Semin Arthritis Rheum 30:217–241, 2001

Harris CM, Hodgkins PR, Kriss A, et al: Familial congenital saccade initiation failure and isolated cerebellar vermis hypoplasia. Dev Med Child Neurol 40:775–779, 1998

Harris CM, Taylor DS, Vellodi A: Ocular motor abnormalities in Gaucher disease. Neuropediatrics 30:289–293, 1999

Hashimoto R, Tanaka Y: Contribution of the supplementary motor area and anterior cingulate gyrus to pathological grasping phenomena. Eur Neurol 40:151–158, 1998

Herzog AG, Edelheit PB, Jacobs AR: Low salivary cortisol levels and aggressive behavior. Arch Gen Psychiatry 58:513–515, 2001

Hopf HC, Muller-Forell W, Hopf NJ: Localization of emotional and volitional facial paresis. Neurology 42:1918–1923, 1992

Ikeda M, Brown J, Holland AJ, et al: Changes in appetite, food preference, and eating habits in frontotemporal dementia and Alzheimer's disease. J Neurol Neurosurg Psychiatry 73:371–376, 2002

Jacks AS, Miller NR: Spontaneous retinal venous pulsation: aetiology and significance. J Neurol Neurosurg Psychiatry 74:7–9, 2003

Jacob A, Cherian PJ, Radhakrishnan K, et al: Emotional facial paresis in temporal lobe epilepsy: its prevalence and lateralizing value. Seizure 12:60–64, 2003

Jacobs AR, Edelheit PB, Coleman AE, et al: Late-onset congenital adrenal hyperplasia: a treatable cause of anxiety. Biol Psychiatry 46:856–859, 1999

Jaspers K: General Psychopathology. Manchester, Manchester University Press, 1963

Jorge R, Robinson RG: Mood disorders following traumatic brain injury. NeuroRehabilitation 17:311–324, 2002

Jorm AF, Christensen H, Korten AE, et al: Memory complaints as a precursor of memory impairment in older people: a longitudinal analysis over 7–8 years. Psychol Med 31:441–449, 2001

Kurowski KM, Blumstein SE, Alexander M: The foreign accent syndrome: a reconsideration. Brain Lang 54:1–25, 1996

Lambert MV: Seizures, hormones and sexuality. Seizure 10:319–340, 2001

Lamberti P, De Mari M, Zenzola A, et al: Frequency of apraxia of eyelid opening in the general population and in patients with extrapyramidal disorders. Neurol Sci 23 (suppl 2):S81–S82, 2002

Lanska DJ, Goetz CG: Romberg's sign: development, adoption, and adaptation in the 19th century. Neurology 55:1201–1206, 2000

Lazar RM, Connaire K, Marshall RS, et al: Developmental deficits in adult patients with arteriovenous malformations. Arch Neurol 56:103–106, 1999

Leigh RJ, Newman SA, Folstein SE, et al: Abnormal ocular motor control in Huntington's disease. Neurology 33:1268–1275, 1983

Lishman WA: Organic Psychiatry: The Psychological Consequences of Cerebral Disorder, 3rd Edition. Malden, MA, Blackwell Science, 1998

Luria AR: Higher Cortical Functions in Man. New York, Basic Books, 1966

McDonald BC, Flashman LA, Saykin AJ: Executive dysfunction following traumatic brain injury: neural substrates and treatment strategies. NeuroRehabilitation 17:333–344, 2002

McGee SR: Evidence-Based Physical Diagnosis. Philadelphia, PA, WB Saunders, 2001

McGrath J, El-Saadi O, Grim V, et al: Minor physical anomalies and quantitative measures of the head and face in patients with psychosis. Arch Gen Psychiatry 59:458–464, 2002

Moldavsky M, Lev D, Lerman-Sagie T: Behavioral phenotypes of genetic syndromes: a reference guide for psychiatrists. J Am Acad Child Adolesc Psychiatry 40:749–761, 2001

Montagna P, Lugaresi E: Agrypnia Excitata: a generalized overactivity syndrome and a useful concept in the neurophysiopathology of sleep. Clin Neurophysiol 113:552–560, 2002

Mori E, Yamadori A: Rejection behaviour: a human homologue of the abnormal behaviour of Denny-Brown and Chambers' monkey with bilateral parietal ablation. J Neurol Neurosurg Psychiatry 52:1260–1266, 1989

Naegele B, Pepin JL, Levy P, et al: Cognitive executive dysfunction in patients with obstructive sleep apnea syndrome (OSAS) after CPAP treatment. Sleep 21:392–397, 1998

Nopoulos P, Berg S, Canady J, et al: Structural brain abnormalities in adult males with clefts of the lip and/or palate. Genet Med 4:1–9, 2002a

Nopoulos P, Berg S, VanDemark D, et al: Cognitive dysfunction in adult males with non-syndromic clefts of the lip and/or palate. Neuropsychologia 40:2178–2184, 2002b

Nutt JG, Marsden CD, Thompson PD: Human walking and higher-level gait disorders, particularly in the elderly. Neurology 43:268–279, 1993

Orient JM, Sapira JD: Sapira's Art and Science of Bedside Diagnosis, 2nd Edition. Philadelphia, PA, Lippincott Williams & Wilkins, 2000

Ovsiew F: Bedside neuropsychiatry: eliciting the clinical phenomena of neuropsychiatric illness, in American Psychiatric Publishing Textbook of Neuropsychiatry and Clinical Neurosciences, 4th Edition. Edited by Yudofsky SC, Hales RE. Washington, DC, American Psychiatric Publishing, 2002, pp 153–198

Ovsiew F, Bylsma FW: The three cognitive examinations. Semin Clin Neuropsychiatry 7:54–64, 2002

Ovsiew F, Utset T: Neuropsychiatry of the rheumatic diseases, in American Psychiatric Publishing Textbook of Neuropsychiatry and Clinical Neurosciences, 4th Edition. Edited by Yudofsky SC, Hales RE. Washington, DC, American Psychiatric Publishing, 2002, pp 813–850

Piazzini A, Canevini MP, Maggiori G, et al: The perception of memory failures in patients with epilepsy. Eur J Neurol 8:613–620, 2001

Pinching AJ: Clinical testing of olfaction reassessed. Brain 100:377–388, 1977

Power C, Selnes OA, Grim JA, et al: HIV Dementia Scale: a rapid screening test. J Acquir Immune Defic Syndr Hum Retrovirol 8:273–278, 1995

Rasmussen P: Persistent mirror movements: a clinical study of 17 children, adolescents and young adults. Dev Med Child Neurol 35:699–707, 1993

Regard M, Landis T: "Gourmand syndrome": eating passion associated with right anterior lesions. Neurology 48:1185–1190, 1997

Rio J, Montalbán J, Pujadas F, et al: Asterixis associated with anatomic cerebral lesions: a study of 45 cases. Acta Neurol Scand 91:377–381, 1995

Rosenbaum A, Hoge SK, Adelman SA, et al: Head injury in partner-abusive men. J Consult Clin Psychol 62:1187–1193, 1994
Russell RW: Supranuclear palsy of eyelid closure. Brain 103:71–82, 1980
Sachdev P, Kruk J: Restlessness: the anatomy of a neuropsychiatric symptom. Aust N Z J Psychiatry 30:38–53, 1996
Sachdev P, Smith JS, Cathcart S: Schizophrenia-like psychosis following traumatic brain injury: a chart-based descriptive and case-control study. Psychol Med 31:231–239, 2001
Salvarani C, Silingardi M, Ghirarduzzi A, et al: Is duplex ultrasonography useful for the diagnosis of giant-cell arteritis? Ann Intern Med 137:232–238, 2002
Sanders RD, Keshavan MS: The neurologic examination in adult psychiatry: from soft signs to hard science. J Neuropsychiatry Clin Neurosci 10:395–404, 1998
Sanders RD, Keshavan MS: Physical and neurologic examinations in neuropsychiatry. Semin Clin Neuropsychiatry 7:18–29, 2002
Saver JL, Greenstein P, Ronthal M, et al: Asymmetric catalepsy after right hemisphere stroke. Mov Disord 8:69–73, 1993
Saygi S, Katz A, Marks DA, et al: Frontal lobe partial seizures and psychogenic seizures: comparison of clinical and ictal characteristics. Neurology 42:1274–1277, 1992
Schott JM, Rossor MN: The grasp and other primitive reflexes. J Neurol Neurosurg Psychiatry 74:558–560, 2003
Seel RT, Kreutzer JS, Rosenthal M, et al: Depression after traumatic brain injury: a National Institute on Disability and Rehabilitation Research Model Systems multicenter investigation. Arch Phys Med Rehabil 84:177–184, 2003
Shahed J, Jankovic J: Re-emergence of childhood stuttering in Parkinson's disease: a hypothesis. Mov Disord 16:114–118, 2001
Shevell M, Ashwal S, Donley D, et al: Practice parameter: evaluation of the child with global developmental delay: report of the Quality Standards Subcommittee of the American Academy of Neurology and The Practice Committee of the Child Neurology Society. Neurology 60:367–380, 2003
Shorr RI, Johnson KC, Wan JY, et al: The prognostic significance of asymptomatic carotid bruits in the elderly. J Gen Intern Med 13:86–90, 1998
Solms M: New findings on the neurological organization of dreaming: implications for psychoanalysis. Psychoanal Q 64:43–67, 1995
Steiner MC, Ward MJ, Ali NJ: Dementia and snoring (case report). Lancet 353:204, 1999

St John P, Montgomery P: Are cognitively intact seniors with subjective memory loss more likely to develop dementia? Int J Geriatr Psychiatry 17:814–820, 2002

Syz H: Recovery from loss of mnemic retention after head trauma. J Gen Psychol 17:355–387, 1937

Szabo K, Gass A, Rossmanith C, et al: Diffusion- and perfusion-weighted MRI demonstrates synergistic lesions in acute ischemic Foix-Chavany-Marie syndrome. J Neurol 249:1735–1737, 2002

Tasman A, Kay J, Lieberman JA: Psychiatry. Philadelphia, PA, WB Saunders, 1997

Tatu L, Moulin T, Monnier G, et al: Unilateral pure thalamic asterixis: clinical, electromyographic, and topographic patterns. Neurology 54:2339–2342, 2000

Tecoma ES, Laxer KD, Barbaro NM, et al: Frequency and characteristics of visual field deficits after surgery for mesial temporal sclerosis. Neurology 43:1235–1238, 1993

Teuber H-L, Liebert RS: Specific and general effects of brain injury in man; evidence of both from a single task. AMA Arch Neurol Psychiatry 80:403–407, 1958

Thompson PD, Marsden CD: Gait disorder of subcortical arteriosclerotic encephalopathy: Binswanger's disease. Mov Disord 2:1–8, 1987

Trixler M, Tenyi T, Csabi G, et al: Minor physical anomalies in schizophrenia and bipolar affective disorder. Schizophr Res 52:195–201, 2001

van Gijn J: The Babinski Sign: A Centenary. Utrecht, Universiteit Utrecht, 1996

Vilensky JA, Gilman S: Positive and negative factors in movement control: a current review of Denny-Brown's hypothesis. J Neurol Sci 151:149–158, 1997

Winkler AS, Reuter I, Harwood G, et al: The frequency and significance of "striatal toe" in parkinsonism. Parkinsonism Relat Disord 9:97–101, 2002

Working Group of the Royal Australasian College of Physicians: Chronic fatigue syndrome. Clinical practice guidelines—2002. Med J Aust 176 (suppl):S23–S56, 2002

Yamanouchi H, Nagura H: Neurological signs and frontal white matter lesions in vascular parkinsonism. A clinicopathologic study. Stroke 28:965–969, 1997

Yates BL, Koran LM: Epidemiology and recognition of neuropsychiatric disorders in mental health settings, in Neuropsychiatry and Mental Health Services. Edited by Ovsiew F. Washington, DC, American Psychiatric Press, 1999, pp 23–67

Zysset S, Huber O, Samson A, et al: Functional specialization within the anterior medial prefrontal cortex: a functional magnetic resonance imaging study with human subjects. Neurosci Lett 335:183–186, 2003

Chapter 2

Neuropsychological Examination of the Psychiatric Patient

Glen E. Getz, M.A.
Mark R. Lovell, Ph.D.

The neuropsychological evaluation plays a significant role in the diagnosis, prognosis, and treatment of neuropsychiatric disorders. A major goal of the neuropsychological assessment is to understand underlying cognitive processes through the quantification of behavior. This approach toward understanding brain-behavior relationships has proved to be useful with a variety of patient populations, including those with dementia, traumatic brain injury, vascular dementia, epilepsy, and developmental disorders. In this chapter we review the applications of neuropsychological assessment in neuropsychiatric populations, methodological issues associated with assessments, and the different types of test batteries typically administered. We also discuss the major neuropsychological instruments that are used to examine various cognitive domains and the ecological validity of neuropsychological assessment. We also briefly address some future considerations in assessment.

Goals of Neuropsychological Examination

The results obtained from a neuropsychological evaluation can be useful in numerous ways. Referral questions range from diagnostic assistance, such as "Does this individual have dementia?"

to questions about functional ability and patient management, such as "Can this person adequately care for himself or herself?" Regardless of the specific purpose of an individual assessment, the three primary goals of all neuropsychological evaluations are to determine an individual's cognitive and behavioral strengths and weaknesses, to interpret the findings from a diagnostic viewpoint, and to recommend viable treatment and rehabilitation resolutions (La Rue 1992). Neuropsychological procedures provide a complement to other medical evaluations. For example, when used in conjunction with quantitative or functional neuroimaging, the neuropsychological assessment enhances the understanding of pathological disturbances of the brain (Howieson and Lezak 2000).

The neuropsychological evaluation is relatively unique in its ability to generate quantifiable information regarding the functional capability of individuals with various psychiatric disorders (Lovell and Nussbaum 1994). In addition, the neuropsychological evaluation provides caretakers with a clearer understanding of the psychosocial consequences of a disease by generating quantitative information regarding cognitive skills. This information can be used in a variety of ways, including deciding on living arrangements, driving ability, and vocational training; determining competency; and making other treatment-related decisions (Acker 1990; Daigneault et al. 2002). This aspect of neuropsychological assessment has become increasingly important because the expected life span has increased and clinicians often have to determine the best course of care for the individual.

Methodological Considerations

A neuropsychological evaluation can be a key component of a patient's treatment in determining the nature and extent of emotional and behavioral problems. It can assist in the clinical diagnostic process and can complement information gathered through other means. However, the utility of these procedures is dependent on the acquisition of test results under controlled conditions. Understanding some important methodological issues involved in the assessment process—specifically the clinical interview and the interpretation of results—is germane to the current chapter.

Clinical Interview Process

The clinical interview provides the basis of the neuropsychological evaluation (Lezak 1995; Sbordone 2000). The clinical interview should produce thorough information regarding the patient's background, including (but not limited to) the patient's chief complaint, confounding factors, educational history, behavioral functioning, medical history, and psychosocial functioning (Sbordone 2000). It also provides the bases for establishing rapport with the patient. During the clinical interview, it is necessary to evaluate the patient's physical limitations, psychological functioning, and approach toward the evaluation. When conducting a neuropsychological evaluation, the clinician should always attempt to incorporate a multimodal examination of sensory abilities (Gregory 1996). Therefore, before administrating the tests it is important to consider whether the patient has hearing or vision deficits. Sensory problems may result in an impaired cognitive profile and could be interpreted as severe cognitive deficits. Furthermore, in the clinical interview the clinician should determine whether the patient is currently taking medication. Many medications have neurocognitive side effects (Glenn and Joseph 1987; Stein and Strickland 1998; Wroblewski et al. 1989), and this factor should always be considered within the context of the neuropsychological evaluation. In certain circumstances it may be best to conduct the testing session when the patient is not currently using the medication so that a true estimate of cognitive abilities can be obtained. For example, when testing a child who is already receiving a stimulant medication, it may be most useful to conduct the test during a period when the child is not taking the medication. Likewise, a patient should never be tested after consuming alcohol. Acute alcohol use can create impairments in short-term memory and executive functioning (Rourke and Loberg 1996). Other physiological factors—such as fatigue, severe headaches, and acute pain—can suppress the performance of an individual in areas of attention, concentration, and working memory.

In addition to drug and medication effects, certain factors need to be constantly reconsidered throughout the course of an evaluation. The motivation and cooperation of the patient are particularly important. To obtain an accurate estimation of cognitive ability, it is important that the patient be encouraged to give his or her best effort on all the tests. If the patient is not motivated to perform at his or her actual level of ability, inaccurate and misleading results are likely to be obtained. Motivation to perform poorly is by no means uncommon and should be evaluated carefully when the secondary gain for poor performance is likely (Binder et al. 2003). Psychological issues, such as anxiety and depression, can also negatively affect cognitive performance and need to be taken into consideration when interpreting the results from a neuropsychological evaluation.

One goal of the evaluation is to estimate premorbid cognitive function to determine if a change in cognition has occurred. In addition to information obtained from reliable secondary sources such as family members and friends, the clinical interview can provide a useful estimation of the patient's premorbid level of cognitive functioning. Another way to estimate premorbid functioning is to use tests that measure the general fund of knowledge, which is typically resistant to brain dysfunction. Intellectual cognitive screening tests, such as the National Adult Reading Test (Nelson 1982) or the North American Adult Reading Test (Spreen and Strauss 1998), are validated tests that are commonly used to determine premorbid intellectual ability (Spreen and Strauss 1998). These tests require the patient to correctly pronounce a list of 50 irregularly spelled words.

Interpretation of Test Results

Although the process of collecting neuropsychological test data represents a standardized and—for the most part—objective process, the interpretation of the data is more subjective (Naugle et al. 1998). There are multiple test-related factors that should be considered when interpreting the results. The clinical neuropsychological evaluation is largely dependent on normative data from an appropriate comparison group. The normative data provide the basis for comparison when determining whether the patient is exhibiting cognitive deficits in relation to others. Deviations below the range of expected performance require interpretation (Lezak 1986, 1995). The analysis should take into consideration the overall pattern of test performance. For example, in an individual who otherwise performs in the above-average or superior range, a single test score that falls in the low-average range may suggest cognitive dysfunction. Although there are no psychiatric conditions that a neuropsychologist might be able to diagnose on the basis of a single test score (Ivnik et al. 2000), the culmination of results from an entire battery of tests is particularly effective in answering the referral question and in aiding in differential diagnosis. It is as important to interpret test results based on the pattern of performance within an individual as it is to compare results for that individual to normative data for each test administered. The following example illustrates this issue:

> A 75-year-old retired English school teacher, who was very active in the community, recently began experiencing functional difficulties in which she would commonly become lost while driving. Her primary-care physician referred her for evaluation to determine whether these difficulties were related to normal aging or early dementia. Her cognitive profile was compared with that of a healthy comparison group of the same age and educational background. Her scores were in the above-average or superior range on tasks of attention, language, and reasoning but were in the low-average and borderline range on tasks of verbal and visual memory. The deviations were significantly below her performance on the other tasks. The cognitive profile and supporting information from the clinical interview were interpreted as mild cognitive impairment. It was noted that such a diagnosis has a strong likelihood of leading to dementia. Six months later, she was reevaluated and exhibited mild word-finding difficulty and increased deficits in verbal and visual memory that were classified well within the impaired range, as she had met criteria for dementia.

This case illustrates the importance of careful examination of the pattern of the patient's performance across multiple cognitive domains, as well as the importance of a clinical understanding of test interpretation beyond the use of a normative comparison group. Likewise, it is also important to use multiple measures that evaluate similar abilities to clarify whether a deficit exists. Multiple tests examining similar aspects of the same cognitive domain may provide corroborative or unique information about the patient's abilities within a given cognitive domain. If an impaired score shows up on only one task, it may represent a clinically insignificant anomaly, or it may be measuring a specific deficit that needs to be examined more thoroughly. Use of multiple tests that examine similar abilities provides for a better understanding of the relative cognitive strengths and weaknesses of the individual. Ultimately, the clinical judgment of the experienced neuropsychologist is necessary for the interpretation of such results.

The utility of a neuropsychological evaluation is dependent on many factors. Conclusions based on an evaluation in which psychometric test scores provide the only information regarding the functioning of a patient should make one wary (Howieson and Lezak 2000). Typically, such an evaluation reflects a narrow understanding of the individual's cognitive and social functioning. It is also important to realize that poor performance on neuropsychological tests does not definitely indicate an underlying brain disorder. Although neuropsychological tests are intended to evaluate neurocognitive functioning, the noncognitive factors mentioned earlier, such as motivation, may play a role in the test outcome.

Approaches to Neuropsychological Assessment

Clinical approaches toward the evaluation of cognitive abilities vary among neuropsychologists, but all approaches constitute attempts to determine whether the patient demonstrates brain-based dysfunction. The main strategies for neuropsychological assessments include fixed batteries of neuropsychological tests and the flexible evaluation tailored toward the individual. In this section, we review the application of these different approaches. We also briefly discuss the utility of mental status evaluations.

Fixed-Battery Approach

With a fixed neuropsychological test battery approach, the same test instruments are utilized in all patients (Kaszniak 1989; Reitan and Wolfson 1993). Such an approach is structured to answer any referral question and to help diagnose any neuropsychiatric conditions that might be present. In this approach, a broad range of abilities are evaluated in every patient through the use of a standardized battery of tests that has previously been validated. Historically, the two most popular fixed neuropsychological batteries have been the Halstead-Reitan Neuropsychological Battery (HRNB) (Reitan and Wolfson 1993) and the Luria-Nebraska Neuropsychological Battery (Incagnoli et al. 1986). It is clear that use of such an approach confers numerous advantages. In particular, the fixed-battery approach provides a comprehensive assessment of multiple cognitive domains, and the test data can be scientifically analyzed for research purposes. However, recent critiques have questioned the practical usefulness of this assessment approach. For example, the fixed battery is labor intensive. Administration of the HRNB may take 6–8 hours, and administration of the Luria-Nebraska Battery takes up to 3 hours. In addition, subtle areas of weakness may be overlooked, whereas aspects of relative cognitive strength may be overevaluated (Howieson and Lezak 2000). Furthermore, given current health care cost restrictions, it has become increasingly difficult to receive authorization to complete such thorough evaluations. Tailoring the evaluation to examine the patient's cognitive functioning within a minimum amount of time and with minimal cost has become a necessary goal for neuropsychologists.

Flexible-Battery Approach

The individualized examination has increased the popularity of the flexible battery. The flexible strategy, also known as hypothesis testing, enables the examiner to select specific tests based on the hypothesis about the etiology and nature of brain dysfunction (Kane 1992; Kaplan 1988; Lezak 1995). With this approach, information obtained throughout the clinical evaluation is used to generate hypotheses regarding possible neuropsychological deficits. The more information obtained through the medical history and clinical interview, the more specific the hypotheses may become. The flexible-battery approach allows the examiner to use the necessary clinical skills to determine which tests are the most beneficial to administer before and during the assessment. Advantages of the flexible approach to evaluation include potentially shorter administration time and the ability to adapt to different patients' needs. However, the amount of information obtained by the neuropsychologist is limited. Such an approach requires extensive clinical training and experience because the interpretation of the test results is both qualitative and quantitative. Furthermore, the flexible approach may not be comprehensive, because deficits that are not readily noticeable may be overlooked whereas obvious difficulties are assessed. The lack of systematic databases also limits the scientific utility of test results by making it difficult to compare results across institutions. However, this individualized approach continues to gain popularity among neuropsychologists.

Mental Status Examination

Regardless of whether the battery used is fixed or flexible, a mental status examination often precedes the neuropsychological evaluation. The purpose of a mental status examination is to provide a brief but accurate description of the patient's functioning in several cognitive areas, including orientation, memory, language, thought content, and insight. A commonly used mental status examination is the Mini-Mental State Exam (Folstein et al. 1975). This 5- to 10-minute screening instrument provides an objective global score of cognitive functioning based on 30 items that briefly measure different cognitive abilities. This instrument is particularly effective when screening for dementia (Ferris 1992). Although mental status examinations provide a quick measure of cognitive functioning as well as additional information from the clinical interview, they should not be used to resolve complicated differential diagnostic issues. A more thorough evaluation of the cognitive domains that are quickly addressed by the mental status examination are often a part of the larger neuropsychological evaluation. Yet a mental status examination may be an excellent screening tool for a physician to use when cognitive impairment is suspected. It can also provide useful preassessment information for a hypothesis-driven test battery.

Major Cognitive Domains and Selected Neuropsychiatric Syndromes

In this section we provide a brief description of the major areas of cognitive functioning covered by neuropsychological evaluations. We include some examples of specific tests used to evaluate different cognitive abilities, as well as some brief diagnostic descriptions obtained from patients' performance on the tests. Table 2–1 presents some typical tests administered for the various cognitive domains. It also lists possible deficits that may be observed from these tests in neuropsychiatric disorders. Specific deficits in different cognitive domains help differentiate neuropsychiatric disorders. This is not an exhaustive list of available tests but rather illustrates some of the more popular test instruments. Several other tests are used to assess cognitive functioning. For a more comprehensive list of tests and description of their administration, the reader is referred to *A Compendium of Neuropsychological Tests*, 2nd Edition, by Spreen and Strauss (1998). The range of possible cognitive deficits found in neuropsychiatric disorders can vary dramatically depending on the severity of the disorder or the location of a lesion. Interpretation of test results requires expertise from qualified professionals.

Intellectual Processes

General intellectual functioning has been defined in numerous ways (Eysenck 1982; Gardner 1983; Terman 1916; Wechsler 1939), but it is broadly considered to be the capacity to learn from experience and to adapt to one's environment (Gregory 1996). The most commonly used set of tests that measures intelligence is the Wechsler Adult Intelligence Scale, 3rd Edition (WAIS-III) (Wechsler 1997a). This battery, which takes 1½–2 hours to admin-

Table 2–1. Cognitive domains, representative neuropsychological tests, and symptoms of neuropsychiatric deficits

Cognitive domain	Tests	Possible performance of neuropsychiatric patients
Intelligence	Wechsler Adult Intelligence Scale, 3rd Edition (WAIS-III) (Wechsler 1997a)	Fund of knowledge typically unaffected; otherwise variable
	Wechsler Intelligence Scale for Children, 3rd Edition (WISC) (Wechsler 1991)	
	Stanford-Binet Intelligence Scale, 4th Edition (Thorndike et al. 1996)	
Memory	Wechsler Memory Scale, 3rd Edition (WMS-III) (Wechsler 1997b)	Recent memory impairment
	California Verbal Learning Test (Delis et al. 1987)	Verbal memory deficit
	Rey-Osterrieth Complex Figure (Osterrieth 1944; Rey 1941; Taylor 1979)	Visual memory deficit
	Benton Visual Retention Test (BVRT) (Benton 1974)	Working memory impairment
	Hopkins Verbal Learning Tests (Brandt 1991)	
	Rey Auditory-Verbal Learning Test (Lezak 1995; Rey 1964)	

Table 2–1. Cognitive domains, representative neuropsychological tests, and symptoms of neuropsychiatric deficits *(continued)*

Cognitive domain	Tests	Possible performance of neuropsychiatric patients
Attention	Digit Span (WAIS-III)	Mental tracking deficits
	Visual Memory Span (WMS-III)	Concentration difficulty
	Continuous Performance Test (Rosvold and Mirsky 1956)	Sustained attention decrement
	Stroop Test (Golden 1978; Stroop 1935)	Divided attention inability
	Cancellation Tests	
	Trail Making Test (Army Individual Test Battery 1944)	
	N-Back Test	
Executive functioning	Category Test (Halstead 1947)	Perseveration
	Wisconsin Card Sorting Test (WCST) (Berg 1948; Heaton 1981)	Lack of planning
	Tower of London Test (Shallice 1982)	Impulsive responding
	Porteus Maze Test (Porteus 1965)	Disorganization
	Stroop Test (Golden 1978; Stroop 1935)	Cognitive inflexibility
	Trail Making Test	Poor judgment/reasoning

Table 2–1. Cognitive domains, representative neuropsychological tests, and symptoms of neuropsychiatric deficits *(continued)*

Cognitive domain	Tests	Possible performance of neuropsychiatric patients
Language	Boston Diagnostic Aphasia Examination (Goodglass and Kaplan 1972)	Poor fluency
	Multilingual Aphasia Examination (Benton and Hamsher 1989)	Anomia
	Reitan-Indiana Aphasia Screening (Reitan and Wolfson 1985)	Word finding difficulty
	Wepman Auditory Discrimination Test (Wepman and Reynolds 1987)	Increase/decrease in output
		Abnormal rate
Motor functioning	Finger Oscillation/Tapping Test (Reitan 1969; Spreen and Strauss 1998)	Limb weakness
	Grooved Pegboard Test (Purdue Research Foundation 1948)	Apraxia
	Purdue Pegboard Test (Purdue Research Foundation 1948)	Impaired fine motor control
	Grip Strength Test (Reitan and Davison 1974)	Decreased motor speed
Visuospatial and visuomotor	Judgment of Line Orientation (Benton et al. 1994)	Spatial disorientation
	Visual Form Discrimination Test (Benton et al. 1994)	Constructional deficits
	Facial Recognition Test (Benton et al. 1994)	Impaired facial recognition
	Block Design (WAIS-III)	Spatial judgment problems
	BVRT and Rey-Osterrieth Complex Figure (copy condition)	

ister, consists of several subtests examining a range of cognitive skills, including abstract solving ability, general fund of knowledge, vocabulary skills, and visuospatial organization. The scores obtained from the WAIS-III can be summed to create an overall intellectual quotient, and the scores can also be separated by performance on the different subscales to create a Verbal intelligence quotient and a Performance intelligence quotient. The WAIS-III also provides index scores in four major areas of cognitive functioning: verbal comprehension, perceptual organization, working memory, and processing speed. Although research to determine the clinical utility of these indices is ongoing, the indices divide the cognitive abilities required for the separate subtests into separate cognitive constructs. A similar version of this test, the Wechsler Intelligence Scale for Children, 3rd Edition (Wechsler 1991), is available for children between ages 6 and 16 years.

Due to time constraints, limitation in a patient's stamina, severity of cognitive impairment, or numerous other reasons, the examiner may not be able to administer the complete WAIS-III. When a brief evaluation of intellectual functioning is desired, a shorter version of the WAIS-III is often administered. There are several suggestions regarding which subscales are the most appropriate (Wechsler 1997a); however, clinicians are often encouraged to administer at least one subscale examining verbal abilities and one subscale measuring performance abilities. An abbreviated version of the test, the Wechsler Abbreviated Scale of Intelligence (WASI) (Wechsler 1999), was recently developed. It includes Vocabulary and Similarities subtests, as well as Block Design and Matrix Reasoning. In the Vocabulary subtest the examinee must define several words, whereas in the Similarities subtest the patient is presented with two items and is asked how they are alike. In the Block Design subtest, the examinee is presented with a picture of a geometric design and must reproduce the design by using colored blocks. In the Matrix Reasoning subtest, the patient is presented with several pictures that are missing a part and is asked to select the correct part from among several choices. Although the WASI is frequently used to save time during the evaluation process, recent research findings have questioned the validity of the WASI compared with the WAIS-III (Axelrod 2002). Future studies should continue to evaluate whether this brief test provides a valid measure of intellectual functioning.

Another intelligence test that merits mentioning is the Stanford-Binet Intelligence Scale, 4th Edition (Thorndike et al. 1996). This scale has 15 subtests that assess ability in four areas: verbal reasoning, abstract/visual reasoning, quantitative reasoning, and short-term memory. Although the original version dates to 1905, this test is less commonly used in current neuropsychological evaluations. However, it remains a useful instrument when measuring cognitive skills in children under age 6 years and in individuals with extremely low functioning.

Memory

The ability to learn new information and to demonstrate retention of previously learned material requires memory function. Memory impairment is one of the most prominent cognitive deficits that occur with neuropsychiatric disorders (Hart and Semple 1990). Memory decline occurs in a variety of neuropsychiatric disorders, such as dementia, traumatic brain injury, schizophrenia, depression, Korsakoff's syndrome, and Huntington's chorea. Memory skills can be classified into several dimensions, including verbal and nonverbal memory, short-term and long-term memory, working memory, recall and recognition, motor memory, and remote memory. Performance within these various areas of memory can help to differentiate diagnosis. For example, a patient who demonstrates impaired free recall with preserved recognition performance is likely to have a retrieval deficit that is characteristic of basal ganglia and frontal-lobe disorders (Cummings 1992). If a patient demonstrates deficits in both free recall and recognition, it is characteristic of pure amnesia. Pure amnesia occurs in specific disorders such as Alzheimer's disease and Korsakoff's syndrome (Kolb and Wishaw 1996).

The battery of tests most commonly used to evaluate memory skills is the Wechsler Memory Scale, 3rd Edition (WMS-III) (Wechsler 1997b). This scale is composed of various tests that measure verbal and visual retention as well as learning through tasks of recall and recognition. They measure immediate and delayed (approximately 30 minutes) memory abilities. The WMS-III includes normative data for individuals of all age groups and has demonstrated excellent validity. Numerous WMS-III scales are discussed throughout this chapter.

Neuropsychological batteries often use a variety of other tests in addition to or instead of the WMS-III to evaluate specific areas of memory. Commonly used assessment procedures to examine different verbal memory processes include list-learning tasks, particularly the Rey Auditory Verbal Learning Test (Lezak 1995; Rey 1964), the Hopkins Verbal Learning Tests (Brandt 1991), and the California Verbal Learning Test (Delis et al. 1987). These tasks present the patient with a long list (12–16) of words with 3–5 repetitions of the list. The patient is required to recite the words back to the examiner, in any order, after each presentation of the list. After presentation of a second distractor list, the patient is asked to repeat the list again. The patient repeats the list from memory after an approximately 20-minute delay. Then the patient is presented with a list of words and is asked whether any of the words were on the original list. Other tasks of verbal memory include reading the patient a story and having the patient repeat it back. This task is a subtest in the WMS-III.

Visuospatial memory is also an important area of assessment. Disruption of spatial memory relative to other tests may indicate right-hemisphere deficits. Tasks that measure spatial memory abilities include reproduction and recall of a complex figure. The Complex Figure Test (Osterrieth 1944; Rey 1941; Taylor 1979) is composed of abstract designs that are presented for an unlimited amount of time while the patient copies the design. After a predetermined delay (e.g., 30–45 minutes), the patient is asked to reproduce the design. In the Benton Visual Retention Test (Benton 1974), examinees are presented with geometric shapes for a brief period and are asked to reproduce the designs from memory. These tests allow for separation of constructional disturbance from impairment of spatial memory.

Remote memory refers to events that occurred during the early years of one's life (La Rue 1992). The assessment of remote memory is difficult because the neuropsychologist is usually uncertain as to whether the patient obtained initial exposure to the information or how much exposure occurred (Craik 1977). In other words, what appears to be a deficit of remote memory may instead represent a fundamental lack of knowledge. Traditional measures of remote memory—such as the Facial Recognition Test (Butters and Albert 1982), the Events Questionnaire (McCarthy and Warrington 1990), and the Remote Memory Test (Beatty et al. 1988)—often assess an individual's ability to recall famous faces or events during different decades of the twentieth century. Another remote memory test is the presidents test, in which the patient is asked to name and recognize the previous six presidents of the United States (Hamsher and Roberts 1985). Research indicates that although remote memory appears to be slightly affected by age, intact elderly patients have demonstrated relatively intact performance (La Rue 1992). Therefore, when remote memory is impaired, it may be a good predictor of underlying neurophysiological deficits.

Attention

From a neuropsychological perspective, attention is a complex cognitive activity that makes it possible to process meaningful stimuli. Attention is an important cognitive skill because it is a prerequisite for successful performance in other cognitive domains (Albert 1981). It is a multifactorial phenomenon; for the purposes of this chapter, attention includes concentration or mental tracking, sustained attention or vigilance, and divided attention.

Auditory attention is commonly assessed with several Wechsler subscales. For example, the Digit Span subtest measures auditory concentration span by assessing the ability of the patient to repeat a string of numbers in both forward and backward order. The backward condition also measures mental tracking. The Visual Memory Span subtest of the WMS-III is the visual equivalent with a motor component. In this subtest the patient is instructed to tap colored boxes on a card in the same order as demonstrated by the administrator. The span tasks increase in sequence, thus measuring sustained attention span limit. Another visual concentration task includes the letter number cancellation tasks (Talland and Schwab 1964). It requires the examinee to cross off designated stimuli on a sheet of paper within a specific amount of time. Results from visual attention tasks may be confounded in patients with visual problems, but they provide an extremely useful measure of attention in patients with hearing problems. Another mental tracking task is the N-Back Test. This is a computerized task in which the patient is instructed to press a button on the keyboard whenever the number presented on the screen is the same as the number that was presented a certain number of steps previously. This task has proved to be particularly useful in neuroimaging studies.

Divided attention is the ability to ignore extraneous information while focusing on specific stimuli. Divided attention is commonly measured by the Stroop Test (Golden 1978; Stroop 1935). This test involves three parts. In the first part, the patient is presented with a list of names of colors, which he or she must read aloud. During the second part, the patient is required to name the colors of a series of X's. In the third part, the patient is presented with a list of names of colors that are printed in different-colored ink and is asked to name the color of the ink, ignoring the word. For example, when the word *green* is printed in blue ink the patient must name the color of the ink (blue), suppressing the tendency to read the word itself. This task measures both executive functioning and divided attention.

Sustained attention, or vigilance, is the ability to maintain attention for an extended period of time. The Continuous Performance Test (Rosvold and Mirsky 1956), a common measure of attention, is now available in several computerized formats (Loong 1988; Nuechterlein 1983). In this test, stimuli (letters or numbers) are presented briefly one at a time on a computer monitor. The patient is to press a button on a joystick or a key on the keyboard every time a specific letter or number appears on the screen. The test sequence can be altered to evaluate the patient's sustained attention abilities over different courses of time. The test results are analyzed to determine when attention deficits occurred during the task.

Executive Functioning

Executive functioning is a broad neuropsychological term that refers to higher-order cognitive processing, such as planning, organization, problem solving, cognitive flexibility, initiation, motivation, judgment, and inhibition. As such, executive functioning is assessed with a variety of neuropsychological measures. Popular executive functioning tasks that measure cognitive flexibility, learning in novel situations, and shifting mental sets include the Wisconsin Card Sorting Test (Berg 1948; Heaton 1981) and the Category Test (Halstead 1947). Other measures of executive functioning are structured to measure planning, initiation, and perseveration (Howieson and Lezak 2000). A commonly used task of mental planning is the Porteus Maze Test (Porteus 1965), which requires the patient to plan and execute an exit out of a series of increasingly complex mazes presented on paper without making any errors. Another test that measures planning ability is the Tower of London Test (Shallice 1982). This test requires the participant to arrange beads onto pegs to resemble a model picture in a specific number of moves. A measure of cognitive flexibility is the Trail Making Test, Part B (Army Individual Test Battery 1944), which is commonly used in many neuropsychological batteries (Lezak 1995; Reitan and Wolfson 1993). In this test, the participants must draw lines between numbers and letters, alternating in consecutive order. This test measures cognitive flexibility and maintaining mental set. Performance on these and other tasks that require novel problem solving, cognitive flexibility, and maintaining mental set is often impaired in patients with neuropsychiatric disorders, particularly when there are deficiencies in the frontal-subcortical circuitry of the brain.

Goldberg et al. (2000) developed a sophisticated battery of executive tasks based on the work of Luria (1973). The Executive Control battery provides detailed information on a number of elements of executive functioning including initiation, perseveration, and praxis.

Language

Deficits in different aspects of language and speech may occur in neuropsychiatric patients. Although language may be affected by normal aging (Albert et al. 1988), a language evaluation provides useful diagnostic information in patients of all ages. Language deficits provide evidence for dysfunction of the left hemisphere. Thus it is necessary to examine the patients' verbal fluency, comprehension, repetition, and reading and writing skills. Neuropsychological testing includes testing for aphasia, which is any severe language deficit caused by brain damage.

There are a number of tests that measure various aspects of language skills. The Multilingual Aphasia Examination (Benton and Hamsher 1989) is a comprehensive battery of tests examining different aspects of language, including spontaneous speech, speech comprehension, repetition, naming, writing, and reading (Benton et al. 1994). The Aphasia Screening Test from the HRNB is another brief assessment of multiple aspects of language, including reading, writing, and calculation skills (Halstead and Wepman 1959). Verbal fluency is commonly measured using the Controlled Oral Word Association Test (Benton et al. 1994) and the Animal Naming subtest of the Boston Diagnostic Aphasia Examination (Goodglass and Kaplan 1972). In both of these tasks the examinee is provided 1 minute to generate as many words as he or she can that begin with a specific letter or that fall under the category of animals. Age-appropriate normative data are used to determine whether fluency ability is normal. A commonly used test that measures confrontational naming abilities is the Boston Naming Test (Kaplan et al. 1983). In this task the patient is asked to name the objects represented by a series of drawings. If the patient is unable to spontaneously name an object, a phonemic cue is provided, followed by a stimulus cue if the patient still cannot name the object.

Motor Processes and Psychomotor Speed

Neuropsychological tests can provide standardized measures of motor functioning in areas of motor strength, motor speed, and complex motor actions. Information regarding motor functioning and reaction time can be diagnostically useful. For example, decreased motor strength or speed may signal a lateralized brain lesion such as a stroke or tumor, or it may occur in other neurological disorders such as Parkinson's disease. On the other hand, the inability to produce complex motor actions could represent apraxia and might suggest that a specific lesion has occurred in the parietal lobes.

Motor speed is assessed through tests of fine motor coordination, such as the Grooved Pegboard Test or the Purdue Pegboard Test (Purdue Research Foundation 1948). In these tasks, the patient must place pins in a board, first with the dominant hand and then with the nondominant hand. It is expected that the patient will perform better with the dominant hand than with the nondominant hand. Absence of this pattern may help to localize the brain lesion to the contralateral hemisphere. The Finger Oscillation Test (Reitan 1969) and other finger-tapping tests (Spreen and Strauss 1998) measure motor speed of the index finger of each hand. The patient is instructed to tap a key as quickly as possible for a certain time interval. Again, better performance is expected with the dominant hand. A motor strength test is the Grip Strength Test (Reitan and Davison 1974). This measure requires the subject to squeeze a dynamometer as hard as possible in the palm of each hand. This task has both diagnostic and prognostic value.

Visuospatial and Visual Constructional Processes

Neuropsychological assessments typically include a number of measures that examine both visuospatial and visual constructional abilities. Visuospatial problems include distortions in the size, distance, and perspective of objects. Visual constructional problems include similar deficits, but the deficits are due to impairments in constructional abilities rather than visuospatial skills. Thus, visuospatial deficits are problems that are not due to an inability to draw a line, but rather are caused by impaired judgment and perception regarding spatial relationships. Motor-free spatial tasks help to differentiate deficits in visuospatial and visuoconstructional deficits. The separation of these related cognitive processes can be useful in the diagnosis and treatment of patients (Howieson and Lezak 2000). Differentiating between these two concepts is most effectively accomplished by comparing the results on constructional tasks to performance on a motor-free spatial task. For example, the Block Design subtest of the WAIS test, as described earlier (see "Intellectual Processes"), evaluates constructional ability. Furthermore, the copy component of the Complex Figure Test also provides adequate information regarding constructional ability. Several motor-free tests measure visuospatial ability. These include Judgment of Line Orientation, Visual Form Discrimination, and the Facial Recognition Test (Benton et al. 1994). In the Judgment of Line Orientation test the patient is presented with a page showing a pattern of lines at the top and a series of line patterns at the bottom. The patient must identify the figure at the bottom of the page that matches the spatial orientation of the figure at the top. In the Visual Form Discrimination Task the patient is presented with a page displaying a design at the top and four designs at the bottom. The patient must determine which design at the bottom of the page is exactly the same as the one at the top. In the Facial Recognition Test the patient is presented with a page showing a picture of a face at the top and six pictures of faces at the bottom. The patient must decide which face or faces at the bottom are the same as the face at the top of the page. It is thought that deficits in the nondominant hemisphere of the brain disturb visuospatial performance more than do deficits in the dominant hemisphere (Benton and Tranel 1993).

Ecological Validity

Generalization and the predictive validity of performance on neuropsychological tests to the patient's ability to function in his or her environment are extremely important issues for neuropsychology. The utility of neuropsychological assessment lies not only in its diagnostic capabilities but also in its ability to provide useful information regarding the patient's ability to perform daily activities (Lovell and Nussbaum 1994). Research indicates that there is a moderate correlation between performance on neuropsychological tests and specific functional skills (Acker 1990). The results from these studies suggest that predictive validity is greater for functional skills that require complex information processing, such as writing a check (McCue et al. 1990). Other research has suggested that specific neuropsychological tests are related to specific functional skills such as grocery shopping ability in patients diagnosed with schizophrenia (Rempfer et al. 2003) and the ability to drive in patients diagnosed with dementia (Daigneault et al. 2002). In addition, performance on neuropsychological tests has been shown to be related to satisfaction in social relationships in patients with mood disorders (Dickerson et al. 2001; Zubieta et al. 2001). Currently, however, many decisions regarding patients' living arrangement and lifestyle are based on neuropsychological performance on traditional neuropsychological measures, which have not been ecologically validated. It remains unclear whether performance on these tests is in fact related to social functioning. Although evaluating community and social functioning in a precise manner remains a challenge (Velligan et al. 2000), the ecological validity of current tests needs to be determined, and new neuropsychological tasks that parallel activities in daily life need to be developed (Zappala et al. 1989).

Future Directions

At the beginning of the twenty-first century, the discipline of neuropsychology continues to expand. As its role in the evaluation of neuropsychiatric patients becomes increasingly important, it is necessary that neuropsychology continues to evolve. The evaluation process must become increasingly efficient while remaining effective. This is likely to occur through the utilization of modern technology.

Computer-Based Neuropsychological Assessment

With the relatively recent advent of the microcomputer, the use of computer-based neuropsychological testing instruments has become increasingly popular and promises to continue to develop in the future (Bleiberg et al. 1998; Schatz and Browndyke 2002). Computerized neuropsychological testing procedures have both distinct advantages and disadvantages compared with more traditional paper-and-pencil assessment procedures that require an examiner to present, score, and interpret the test data. First and foremost, computerized testing programs allow for standardized presentation of neuropsychological stimuli and therefore minimize differences in test results that might result from differences in test administration. Because the stimuli are delivered in precisely the same manner and administration and scoring of the tests follow a computer-based algorithm, administration and scoring error can be strictly controlled and minimized. This is particularly important when a patient might be evaluated by different neuropsychologists or neuropsychological laboratories, using varying administration and scoring approaches. Second, computers are capable of greater precision regarding cognitive processing speed and reaction time than are traditional approaches that are based on the use of a stopwatch. This, in turn, has allowed neuropsychologists to become increasingly sophisticated in detecting subtle neurocognitive dysfunction such as that occurring after mild traumatic brain injury (Lovell et al. 2003) or as a result of attention-deficit disorder (Barkley et al. 2001). Third, computer-based approaches to neuropsychological assessment allow for minimization of practice effects that naturally occur when an individual is exposed to the same test on multiple occasions. In addition, stimuli can be randomized by the computer, creating a nearly infinite array of test forms. This capacity, in turn, creates the potential for the accurate measurement of subtle deficits in cognitive processes as a result of therapeutic intervention.

One currently popular application of automated neuropsychological testing procedures that has been well researched is in the evaluation of child and adolescent athletes before their return to the playing field after a concussion. For instance, Lovell and his colleagues (Lovell et al. 2003; Maroon et al. 2000) created the ImPACT computer-based program and implemented it in more than 300 high schools and colleges nationally. Through the use of this program, athletes who have had concussions have been found to experience mild neurocognitive dysfunction for up to a week after injury. Another example of the implementation of computer-based testing procedures involves the tracking of improvement in attentional processes after administration of psychostimulant or other medication in children with attention-deficit disorder (Barkley et al. 2001).

Another evolving technology that may prove to be beneficial in assessment is virtual-reality testing. Virtual-reality testing is the human-computer interaction that allows a person to become engaged in a computer-generated environment by using a head-mounted unit. Tracking devices report information to a computer, which continually updates the images presented to the head-mounted unit. Although such technology remains relatively new in the field of neuropsychology, it has been used successfully in other medical fields (Cosman et al. 2002; Stava 1995). Such an approach appears to have the possibility of increasing the ecological validity of neuropsychological testing by evaluating cognitive functioning within a dynamic environment (Schultheis et al. 2002).

Although computer-based approaches to neuropsychological assessment have numerous potential advantages over traditional neuropsychological assessment instruments, there are also potential disadvantages. First, the utilization of computerized procedures by undertrained individuals may lead to spurious test results. In addition, the use of computer technology may lead to reductions in face-to-face interaction with a clinician, resulting in a different experience for the examinee (Honaker 1988) and potentially resulting in misdiagnosis (Space 1981). There are also likely to be subtle technical differences between individual microcomputers and computer systems (Schatz and Zillmer 2003).

As computer technology continues to develop, other applications will no doubt be developed, researched, and implemented in clinical populations. In addition to the above-mentioned advantages of computer-based neuropsychological testing, computers potentially have the advantage of facilitating research by automatically producing data-based information for study and analysis. Finally, with proper supervision, computer-based procedures represent an economical way of acquiring neuropsychological test information in an era in which the health care dollar continues to shrink (French and Beaumont 1987).

References

Acker MB: A review of the ecological validity of neuropsychological tests, in The Neuropsychology of Everyday Life: Assessment and Basic Competencies (Foundations of Neuropsychology, vol 2). Edited by Tupper DE, Cicerone KD. Boston, MA, Kluwer, 1990, pp 19–55

Albert MS: Geriatric neuropsychology. J Consult Clin Psychol 49:835–850, 1981

Albert MS, Moss MB: Geriatric Neuropsychology. New York, Guilford, 1988

Army Individual Test Battery: Manual of Directions and Scoring. Washington, DC, War Department, Adjutant General's Office, 1944

Axelrod BN: Validity of the Wechsler Abbreviated Scale of Intelligence and other very short forms of estimating intellectual functioning. Assessment 9:17–23, 2002

Barkley RA, Edwards G, Laneri M, et al: Executive functioning, temporal discounting, and sense of time in adolescents with attention deficit hyperactivity disorder (ADHD) and oppositional defiant disorder (ODD). J Abnorm Child Psychol 29:541–556, 2001

Beatty WW, Goodkin DE, Monson N, et al: Anterograde and retrograde amnesia in patients with chronic progressive multiple sclerosis. Arch Neurol 45:1113–1119, 1988

Benton AL: The Revised Visual Retention Test, 4th Edition. New York, Psychological Corporation, 1974

Benton AL, Hamsher K: Multilingual Aphasia Examination, 2nd Edition. Iowa City, IA, AJA Associates, 1989

Benton AL, Tranel D: Visuoperceptual, visuospatial and visuoconstructional disorders, in Clinical Neuropsychology. Edited by Heilman KM, Valenstein E. New York, Oxford University Press, 1993, pp 461–497

Benton AL, Silcan AG, Hamsher K de S, et al: Contributions to Neuropsychological Assessment. New York, Oxford University Press, 1994

Berg GE: A simple objective test of measuring flexibility in thinking. J Gen Psychol 39:15–22, 1948

Binder LM, Kelly MP, Villanueva MR: Motivation and neuropsychological test performance following mild head injury. J Clin Exp Neuropsychol 25:420–430, 2003

Bleiberg J, Halpern EL, Reeves D, et al: Future direction for the neuropsychological assessment of sports related concussion. J Head Trauma Rehabil 13:36–44, 1998

Brandt J: The Hopkins Verbal Learning Test: development of a new memory test with six equivalent forms. Clin Neuropsychol 5:125–142, 1991

Butters N, Albert MS: Process underlying failures to recall remote events, in Human Memory and Amnesia. Edited by Cermak BS. Hillsdale, NJ, Lawrence Erlbaum, 1982

Cosman PH, Cregan PC, Martin CJ, et al: Virtual reality simulators: current status in acquisition and assessment of surgical skills. Aust N Z J Surg 72:30–34, 2002

Craik FIM: Age differences in human memory, in Handbook of the Psychology of Aging. Edited by Birren JE, Schaie KW. New York, Van Nostrand Reinhold, 1977, pp 384–420

Cummings JL: Neuropsychiatric aspects of Alzheimer's disease and other dementing illnesses, in The American Psychiatric Press Textbook of Neuropsychiatry, 2nd Edition. Edited by Yudofsky SC, Hales RE. Washington, DC, American Psychiatric Press, 1992, pp 605–620

Daigneault G, Joly P, Frigon JY: Executive functions in the evaluation of accident risk of older drivers. J Clin Exp Neuropsychol 24:221–238, 2002

Delis D, Kramer JH, Kaplan E, et al: The California Verbal Learning Test–Adult Version. San Antonio, TX, Psychological Corporation, 1987

Dickerson FB, Sommerville J, Origoni AE, et al: Outpatients with schizophrenia and bipolar I disorder: do they differ in their cognitive and social functioning? Psychiatry Res 102:21–27, 2001

Eysenck HJ: A Model for Intelligence. Heidelberg, Springer-Verlag, 1982

Ferris SH: Alzheimer's disease. Diagnosis by specialists: psychological testing. Acta Neurol Scand Suppl 139:32–35, 1992

Folstein MF, Folstein SE, McHugh PR: Mini-Mental State: a practical method for grading the cognitive state of patients for the clinician. J Psychiatr Res 12:189–198, 1975

French CC, Beaumont JG: The reaction of psychiatric patients to computerized assessment. Br J Clin Psychol 26:267–277, 1987

Gardner H: Frames of Mind: The Theory of Multiple Intelligence. New York, Basic Books, 1983

Glenn MB, Joseph AB: The use of lithium for behavioral and affective disorders after traumatic brain injury. J Head Trauma Rehabil 2:68–76, 1987

Goldberg E, Podell K, Bilder RM, et al: The Executive Control Battery. Melbourne, Australia, PsychPress, 2000

Golden CJ: The Stroop Color and Word Test: A Manual for Clinical and Experimental Use. Chicago, IL, Stoelting, 1978

Goodglass H, Kaplan E: Assessment of Aphasia and Related Disorders. Philadelphia, PA, Lea & Febiger, 1972

Gregory RJ: Neuropsychological and geriatric assessment, in Psychological Testing: History Principles, and Applications, 2nd Edition. Needham Heights, MA, Allyn & Bacon, 1996, pp 332–385

Halstead WC: Brain and Intelligence. Chicago, IL, University of Chicago Press, 1947

Halstead WC, Wepman JM: The Halstead-Wepman Aphasia Screening Test. J Speech Hear Disord 14:9–15, 1959

Hamsher KD, Roberts RJ: Memory for recent U.S. presidents in patients with cerebral disease. J Clin Exp Neuropsychol 7:1–13, 1985

Hart S, Semple JM: Brain Damage, Behaviour and Cognition: Neuropsychology and the Dementias. Bristol, PA, Taylor & Francis, 1990

Heaton RK: Wisconsin Card Sorting Test Manual. Odessa, FL, Psychological Assessment Resources, 1981

Honaker L: The equivalency of computerized and conventional MMPI administrations: a critical review. Clin Psychol Rev 8:561–577, 1988

Howieson DB, Lezak MD: The neuropsychological evaluation, in The American Psychiatric Textbook of Neuropsychiatry and Clinical Neurosciences, 4th Edition. Edited by Yudofsky SC, Hales RE. Washington, DC, American Psychiatric Press, 2000, pp 217–244

Incagnoli T, Goldstein G, Golden CJ: Neuropsychological Test Batteries. New York, Plenum, 1986

Ivnik RJ, Smith GE, Petersen RC, et al: Diagnostic accuracy of four approaches to interpreting neuropsychological test data. Neuropsychology 14:163–177, 2000

Kane RL: Standardized and flexible batteries in neuropsychology: an assessment update. Neuropsychol Rev 2:281–339, 1992

Kaplan E: A process approach to neuropsychological assessment, in Clinical Neuropsychological and Brain Function: Research, Measurement and Practice. Edited by Boll T, Bryant BK. Washington, DC, American Psychological Association, 1988, pp 125–167

Kaplan EF, Goodglass H, Weintraub S: The Boston Naming Test. Philadelphia, PA, Lea & Febiger, 1983

Kaszniak AW: Psychological assessment of the aging individual, in Handbook of the Psychology of Aging. Edited by Birren JE, Schaie KW. San Diego, CA, Academic Press, 1989, pp 427–445

Kolb B, Wishaw IQ: Fundamentals of Human Neuropsychology, 4th Edition. New York, WH Freeman, 1996

La Rue A: Aging and Neuropsychological Assessment. New York, Plenum, 1992

Lezak MD: An individual approach to neuropsychological assessment, in Clinical Neuropsychology. Edited by Logue PE, Schaer JM. Springfield, IL, Charles C Thomas, 1986, pp 29–49

Lezak MD: Neuropsychological Assessment, 3rd Edition. New York, Oxford University Press, 1995

Loong WK: The Continuous Performance Test. San Luis Obispo, CA, Wang Neuropsychological Laboratory, 1988

Lovell MR, Nussbaum PD: Neuropsychological assessment, in The American Psychiatric Press Textbook of Geriatric Neuropsychiatry. Edited by Coffey CE, Cummings JL. Washington, DC, American Psychiatric Press, 1994, pp 129–144

Lovell MR, Collins MW, Iversion GL, et al: Recovery from mild concussion in high school athletes. J Neurosurg 98:296–301, 2003

Luria AR: The Working Brain: An Introduction to Neuropsychology. Translated by Haigh B. New York, Basic Books, 1973

Maroon JC, Lovell MR, Collins MW, et al: Cerebral concussion in athletes: evaluation and neuropsychological testing. Neurosurgery 47:659–669, 2000

McCarthy RA, Warrington EK: Cognitive Neuropsychology: A Clinical Introduction. San Diego, CA, Academic Press, 1990

McCue M, Rogers J, Goldstein G: Relationships between neuropsychological and functional assessment in elderly neuropsychiatric patients. Rehabil Psychol 3:91–95, 1990

Naugle R, Cullum CM, Bigler ED: Neuropsychological assessment, in Introduction to Clinical Neuropsychology: A Casebook. Austin, TX, PRO-ED, 1998, pp 1–18

Nelson HE: The National Adult Reading Test (NART): Test Manual. Windsor, United Kingdom, NFER-Nelson, 1982

Nuechterlein KH: Signal detection in vigilance tasks and behavioral attributes among offspring of schizophrenia mothers and among hyperactive children. J Abnorm Psychol 92:4–28, 1983

Osterrieth PA: Le test de copie d' une figure complexe. Archives de Psychologie 30:306–356, 1944

Porteus SD: Porteus Maze Test: Fifty Years' Application. Palo Alto, CA, Pacific Books, 1965

Purdue Research Foundation: Examiners Manual for the Purdue Pegboard. Chicago, IL, Science Research Associates, 1948

Reitan RM: Manual for the Administration of Neuropsychological Test Batteries for Adults and Children. Indianapolis, IN, Author, 1969

Reitan RM, Davison LA: Clinical Neuropsychology: Current Status and Applications. New York, Winston-Wiley, 1974
Reitan RM, Wolfson D: The Halstead-Reitan Neuropsychological Test Battery: Theory and Clinical Interpretation, 2nd Edition. Tucson, AZ, Neuropsychology Press, 1993
Rempfer MV, Hamera EK, Brown CE, et al: The relations between cognition and the independent living skill of shopping in people with schizophrenia. Psychiatry Res 117:103–112, 2003
Rey A: L'examen psychologique dans les cas d'encephalopathie traumatique. Archives de Psychologie 28:286–340, 1941
Rey A: L'Examen Clinique En Psychologie. Paris, Press Universitaires de France, 1964
Rosvold HE, Mirsky AF: A continuous performance test of brain damage. J Consult Psychol 20:343–350, 1956
Rourke SB, Loberg T: The neuropsychological correlates of alcoholism, in Neuropsychological Assessment of Neuropsychiatric Disorders, 2nd Edition. Edited by Grant I, Adams KM. New York, Oxford University Press, 1996, pp 423–485
Sbordone RJ: The assessment interview in clinical neuropsychology, in Neuropsychological Assessment in Clinical Practice. Edited by Groth-Maranat G. New York, Wiley, 2000, pp 94–126
Schatz P, Browndyke J: Applications of computer-based neuropsychological assessment. J Head Trauma Rehabil 17:395–410, 2002
Schatz P, Zillmer EA: Computer-based assessment of sports-related concussion. Appl Neuropsychol 10:42–47, 2003
Schultheis MT, Himelstein J, Rizzo AA: Virtual reality and neuropsychology: upgrading the current tools. J Head Trauma Rehabil 17:378–394, 2002
Shallice T: Specific impairments of planning. Philos Trans R Soc Lond B Biol Sci 298:199–209, 1982
Space LG: The computer as psychometrician. Behavior Research Methods and Instrumentation 13:595–606, 1981
Spreen O, Strauss E: A Compendium of Neuropsychological Tests, 2nd Edition. New York, Oxford University Press, 1998
Stava RM: Medical applications in virtual reality. J Med Syst 19:275–280, 1995
Stein RA, Strickland TL: A review of the neuropsychological effects of commonly used prescription medications. Arch Clin Neuropsychol 13:259–284, 1998
Stroop JR: Studies of interference in serial verbal reactions. J Exp Psychol 18:643–662, 1935

Talland GA, Schwab RS: Performance with multiple sets in Parkinson's disease. Neuropsychologia 2:45–53, 1964

Taylor LB: Psychological assessment of neurosurgical patients, in Functional Neurosurgery. Edited by Rasmussen T, Marino R. New York, Raven, 1979

Terman LM: The Measurement of Intelligence. Boston, MA, Houghton Mifflin, 1916

Thorndike RL, Hagen E, Sattler J: Stanford-Binet Intelligence Scale, 4th Edition. Itasca, IL, Riverside, 1996

Velligan DI, Bow-Thomas CC, Mahurin RK, et al: Do specific neurocognitive deficits predict specific domains of community function in schizophrenia? J Nerv Ment Dis 188:518–524, 2000

Wechsler D: The Measurement of Adult Intelligence. Baltimore, MD, Williams & Wilkins, 1939

Wechsler D: WISC-III Manual. Wechsler Intelligence Scale for Children—III. New York, Psychological Corporation, 1991

Wechsler D: WAIS-III. Administration and Scoring Manual. San Antonio, TX, Psychological Corporation, 1997a

Wechsler D: WMS-III. Administration and Scoring Manual. San Antonio, TX, Psychological Corporation, 1997b

Wechsler D: Wechsler Abbreviated Scale of Intelligence (WASI) Manual. San Antonio, TX, Psychological Association, 1999

Wepman JM, Reynolds WM: Wepman's Auditory Discrimination Test, 2nd Edition. Los Angeles, CA, Western Psychological Services, 1987

Wroblewski BA, Glenn MB, Whyte J, et al: Carbamazepine replacement of phenytoin, phenobarbital and primidone in rehabilitation setting: effects on seizure control. Brain Inj 3:149–156, 1989

Zappala G, Martini E, Crook T, et al: Ecological memory assessment in normal aging: a preliminary report on an Italian population. Clin Geriatr Med 5:583–594, 1989

Zubieta JK, Huguelet P, O'Neil R, et al: Cognitive function in euthymic bipolar I disorder. Psychiatry Res 102:9–20, 2001

Chapter 3

Electrophysiological Testing

Nashaat N. Boutros, M.D.
Frederick A. Struve, Ph.D.

Laboratory tests are an essential part of the practice of modern medicine. Laboratory tests can be used to establish diagnoses, to provide supportive evidence for one diagnosis versus another on a differential diagnostic list, or to rule out a particular diagnostic possibility. Thorough knowledge of the proper indications for requesting a particular test, its drawbacks if any (including any danger to the patient), and the clinical meaning of the results are essential for a clinician to skillfully utilize the test in managing a specific patient. When tests are used out of context, they can hinder the diagnostic and treatment process and increase the cost of management unnecessarily (Steffens and Krishnan 2003). There are essentially two types of diagnostic tests (Feinstein 1977). The first type is dichotomous or pathognomonic tests (the results show the disease to be either present or absent). A good example of this type of test is HIV testing. Of course, dichotomous tests can have different levels of sensitivity, but they remain yes-or-no (positive or negative) tests. The second type of laboratory tests, surrogate tests, produce a range of results from which low or high numbers can be used to infer the presence of a disorder. A good example of this type of test is blood cholesterol measurement. With the second type of test the clinical interpretation is more complicated because it requires knowledge about the relationships between different levels of the particular variable measured; race, gender, and age effects; and the prevalence of the disease in question in a particular population. In general, for a test to be clinically useful, the technical aspects of the test should be established (it is best if they are standardized across laboratories), the sensitivity and specificity of the test in detecting a certain disorder should be known, the actual value of the test in clinical settings should be established, and the cost-benefit ratio of the test should also be known (see Steffens and Krishnan 2003 for more in-depth discussion of this topic).

The process of developing a laboratory diagnostic test has a number of stages. The process begins when a biological variable in a particular patient population is observed to be deviant from measurements taken in healthy control subjects. Replication of the finding by the same or collaborating groups is important, but confirmation by independent groups is essential for this particular test to move into the next stage of development. The second stage involves a better understanding of the sensitivity and specificity of the biological marker for identifying a certain group. During this stage the clinical characteristics of the patient group identified by the test are usually further delineated. Because of the heterogeneous nature of psychiatric disorders, it would be naïve to expect any one biological test to be able to identify all patients who fit into a certain DSM-based category (e.g., schizophrenia). It is much more likely that a particular test will be able to identify one or more subgroups within these categories. Defining the clinical characteristics of the subgroup that is identifiable by a particular test would be very important for the test to be considered for clinical use. At this stage the test would be considered promising for development as a diagnostic test. The next stage then includes studies designed specifically to examine the usefulness of the test in clinical settings. The two most important variables at this stage are the choice of patient control groups (these should be groups of patients with diagnoses that commonly appear on the differential diagnostic lists of the target disorder) and the choice of the gold standard or reference test. This is the standard against which the test being developed will be measured. Tests that prove capable of significantly contributing to the differential diagnostic process should then move to the final stage of large multicenter clinical trials. These multicenter trials should pave the way toward standardization of the laboratory procedures used to conduct the test and should provide data on the cost-effectiveness of the test and its impact on the socioeconomic well-being of tested patients.

Special Problems With Laboratory Testing in Neuropsychiatric Disorders

Dichotomous tests are used in psychiatry. The main reason for using such tests is to rule out organicity. This usually means excluding a medical or neurological cause for the presenting symptoms. For example, a person presenting with recent-onset personality change at age 50 may be harboring a space-occupying lesion in the frontal lobe. A computed tomographic (CT) scan or a magnetic resonance imaging (MRI) study can confirm or exclude this possibility. Similarly, an individual with seizurelike episodes who is suspected of having psychogenic rather than epileptic attacks could benefit from a simultaneous electroencephalogram (EEG) and video monitoring of the seizure. A normal EEG during what seems to be a generalized tonic-clonic seizure is usually taken as strong evidence for the episodes to be of a psychogenic origin. Another good example is the presence of thyroid abnormalities in a patient presenting with symptoms that can be explained by hypothyroidism or hyperthyroidism. On the other hand, none of these tests are of great use in differentiating among the so-called functional psychiatric disorders. A number of neuroendocrine, imaging, and electrophysiological tests are beginning to emerge as possible tools that may help clinicians by improving the diagnostic accuracy in differentiating among functional disorders. Most of these biological tests remain in an early phase of development (e.g., showing promising findings) as outlined earlier. A significant problem with all these tests is a strong tendency for them to be released for clinical practice before all (or even the majority) of the variables that are necessary for clinical usefulness (as outlined earlier) have been worked out. The premature release of such tests could lead to disappointment among the medical community and could result in the premature abandonment of the test, as occurred with the dexamethasone suppression test. Premature release could also lead to a severe backlash when limitations of the test—particularly when it is applied in a noncontrolled setting such as in private clinical practice—become apparent and could result in serious delay in the progress of the proper development and evaluation of the test. A good example of the latter is the premature marketing of quantitative electroencephalography to physicians with no training in electrophysiological methodology (Nuwer 1989). However, during the past decade, more than 500 papers on electroencephalography and quantitative electroencephalography have reported well-designed studies, and an overview of this literature reveals numerous consistent quantitative electroencephalographic findings among psychiatric patients within the same DSM diagnostic categories (Hughes and John 1999). In the following section brief descriptions of such electrophysiological procedures are presented, followed by brief discussions of their usefulness or potential (as of the current state of knowledge) in specific clinical situations.

Finally, the issue of the gold standard is particularly problematic in psychiatry. Whereas in most medical conditions tissue diagnosis is possible, allowing the investigators to have a high degree of certainty regarding the presence or absence of the disorder being tested, such a standard does not exist in psychiatry. Instead, psychiatry relies on the best-estimate diagnosis. This standard is based on agreement among a number of experts. Studies by Roy et al. (1997) and by Leckman et al. (1982) showed that when basing diagnoses solely on clinical data, using the best available expertise and a multilevel evaluation to arrive at a consensus best-estimate diagnosis, the agreement coefficient (κ) will not exceed 0.69. For a test to be of clinical usefulness it must be demonstrated that it will incrementally improve the diagnostic ability of the clinician. The degree of improvement necessary for a test to be considered cost-effective is also a complicated question that depends on the particular disorder and the specific clinical situation. Finally, methodology for demonstrating the ability of a test to improve diagnostic accuracy in psychiatry has not been well developed.

Electrophysiological Testing Modalities

Electrophysiological testing is basically noninvasive and is relatively inexpensive. These attributes, combined with the demonstrated prevalence of electrophysiological abnormalities in almost every psychiatric condition, make these modalities both suitable and promising for becoming clinically useful adjuncts to the processes of differential diagnosis, overall prognosis, and even prediction of response to various forms of somatic and psychotherapeutic interventions. In this chapter we focus mainly on how the various electrophysiological testing methods can inform the differential diagnostic process in neuropsychiatric practices. Throughout the discussion, significant emphasis is placed on the routine EEG, because it is the most widely available test. We begin with a brief introduction to the different modalities discussed in the chapter.

Standard EEG

The term *standard EEG* refers to the raw EEG recorded from the scalp and visually inspected by an experienced electroencephalographer. The term *standard* applies to both paper and digital EEGs. The standard EEG is widely available and is relatively inexpensive. For the EEG to be maximally useful, it is crucial that the clinician ordering the test be familiar with the limitations of the test and with the general implications of the different abnormalities that can be detected through an EEG. Two types of electroencephalographic abnormalities can generally be looked for: paroxysmal activity, indicating episodic and unpredictable abnormal neuronal discharges; and nonparoxysmal activity, characterized by slowing of the normal intrinsic rhythms of the brain. Both types of abnormalities can be seen either diffusely (indicating a more generalized pathological process) or focally (indicating a localized pathological process). Furthermore, it is possible for both paroxysmal and nonparoxysmal abnormalities to coexist in the same electroencephalographic tracing.

The most frequent reason for an electroencephalographic referral is to exclude a general medical condition (as in delirium) or a specific neurological problem (e.g., epilepsy) as a cause or a contributing factor for the presenting symptomatology. DSM-IV and DSM-IV-TR (American Psychiatric Association 1994, 2000) require that a general medical condition be excluded before the differential diagnostic process can proceed, and the exclusion of a general medical condition is given as the first step in the differential diagnostic process. However, the DSM system does not give clear guidance on how that exclusion should be accomplished. The use of routine batteries of tests to exclude medical conditions seems unjustifiable in the current cost-conscious environment. Instead, clinicians will need to rely on the two main red flags to trigger organic workups: unusual presentations and atypical age at onset. Inui et al. (1998) emphasized an atypical clinical presentation as the most important factor in deciding to initiate an electroencephalographic evaluation. Secondary red flags might include an unexpected adverse response to treatment presumed to be effective for a certain condition or an absence of benefit even though compliance with the treatment regimen has been verified. Finally, the care of a geriatric patient should be accompanied by a higher index of suspicion for the existence of covert organic variables contributing to the clinical picture.

A chapter on neuropsychiatric electrophysiology would be incomplete without mention of so-called controversial sharp waves or spikes. For a more thorough discussion, the reader is referred to Boutros and Struve (2002). Four electroencephalographic patterns are consistently observed to be more prevalent in psychiatric populations than in control populations of either healthy subjects or nonpsychiatric patients. The four patterns are *14- and 6-per-second positive spikes* (also called stenoids) (Figure 3–1), *rhythmic midtemporal discharges* (originally called psychomotor variants), *small sharp spikes* (also called benign epileptiform transients of sleep), and *6-per-second spike and wave* (also referred to as the 6-per-second spike-wave phantom because of its low-voltage appearance). Despite the substantially increased prevalence of these patterns in psychiatric patients compared with nonpsychiatric control subjects, defining the exact neurobiological basis and clinical correlates of each of these patterns has proved to be an elusive goal. Recent advances in diagnostic capabilities, the ability to define symptom clusters within a particular diagnosis, and the advancing fields of source localization and dense electrode array EEGs have not yet been applied to examination of these phenomena. Although these patterns have sometimes been referred to in the literature as epileptiform, it should be noted that with the possible exception of small sharp spikes (Hughes and Gruener 1984; Saito et al. 1987), none of the patterns have been shown to predictably correlate with seizure disorders. The diagnostic value of these waveforms remains in the first phase of development as diagnostic markers. Nonetheless, the presence of any of these waveforms in a patient who is not responding to standard treatment raises the possibility that a trial of an anticonvulsant may be useful.

Limitations of the Standard EEG

Electroencephalography is burdened by several constraints that place certain limitations on the information it can provide. These constraints, which are extensively discussed elsewhere (Struve 1985), include the following:

- *Limited coverage.* Vast areas of brain tissue are inaccessible to measurement by external scalp electrodes.
- *Limited sensitivity.* Skin, skull, dura, and brain tissue impose varying degrees of impedance between the source of the electrical discharge and the scalp electrodes.
- *Time sampling limitations.* Many important electroencephalographic abnormalities are paroxysmal or episodic in their appearance.
- *Fluctuating substrate physiology.* Numerous variables from pharmacological agents and drugs of abuse to endocrinological and metabolic factors can fluctuate, producing EEGs that may be normal at one time and abnormal at another. A summary of the incidence of electroencephalographic abnormalities associated with selected antipsychotic agents is shown in Figure 3–2.
- *Nonspecificity of results.* The electrical activity of the brain can respond to stimuli or insult only by becoming higher or lower in either frequency or voltage (or some combination of the two); therefore different causes can produce identical electroencephalographic abnormalities.

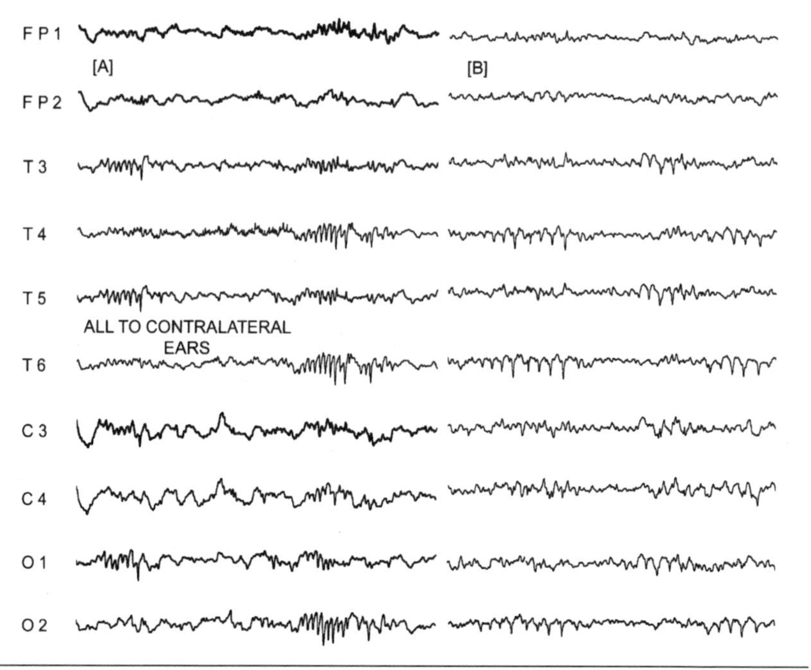

Figure 3–1. Independent left and right midtemporal–posterior temporal–occipital 14- and 6-per-second positive spikes.
A: Electroencephalographic tracing from a 13-year-old girl displaying 14 spikes per second. **B:** Electroencephalographic tracing from a 24-year-old man displaying the 6-spikes-per-second variety. An electroencephalogram may contain either variety alone or a combination of the two.
Source. Reprinted from Boutros NN, Struve FA: "Applied Electrophysiology," in *Kaplan and Sadock's Comprehensive Textbook of Psychiatry,* 8th Edition. Edited by Sadock BJ, Sadock VA. Baltimore, MD, Lippincott Williams & Wilkins, in press. Used with permission.

The use of electroencephalography for assessing mass lesions has two drawbacks. First, very slow-growing lesions may not cause many electroencephalographic changes, particularly if the lesions are small or are not located near the cortex. Second, in uncooperative patients, eye movement artifacts could mask frontally located abnormal activity. An alert technician can avoid this pitfall by applying eye leads for patients exhibiting increased eye movement or by gently taping cotton-ball eye pads over the closed eyelids to reduce eye movement (particularly blinks).

For a number of reasons, EEGs may sometimes fail to detect

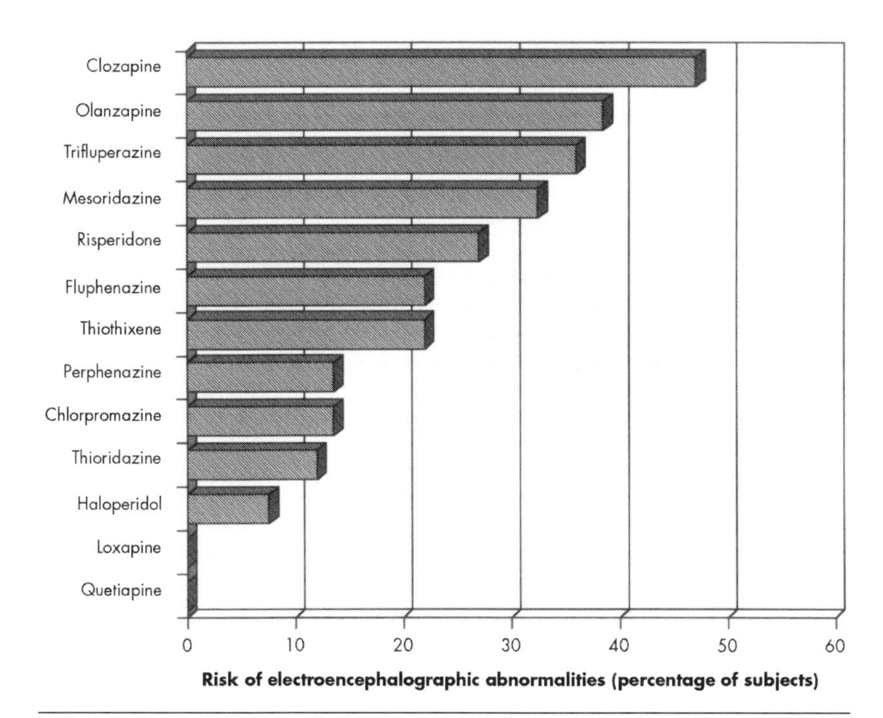

Figure 3–2. Graph showing the relative risk of electroencephalographic abnormalities with specific antipsychotic agents among 293 hospitalized patients.

Source. Reprinted from Centorrino F, Price BH, Tuttle M, et al.: "EEG Abnormalities During Treatment With Typical and Atypical Antipsychotics." *American Journal of Psychiatry* 159:109–115, 2002. Used with permission.

epileptiform discharges in patients with seizure disorders. Except in extreme cases, epileptiform activity is usually not consistently present throughout the entire recording, and a brief EEG may miss activity that would be seen with a longer tracing. Furthermore, some paroxysmal discharges are dependent on drowsy or light-sleep activation, and a normal EEG that does not contain sleep may constitute a false negative. When paroxysmal discharges are very infrequent, serial EEGs must be administered to increase the possibility of a positive finding, and this drives up the cost of the patient's workup. Deep or medial temporal lobe epileptiform discharges may also be undetectable by a surface EEG.

These constraints and limitations have practical relevance. Most important for the practitioner is the fact that most electroencephalographic abnormalities are largely nonspecific, and in such instances the nature of the exact pathological process underlying the electroencephalographic changes cannot be determined based on the EEG alone. Of course, all general principles have their exceptions. Direct confirmation of petit mal status or complex partial seizure status can be made at the moment of EEG recording, and there are a few electroencephalographic waveforms that appear to be fairly specific to certain medical conditions (e.g., triphasic waves with severe liver disease).

Finally, for an electroencephalographic evaluation to be considered adequate, the clinical question that led to the electroencephalographic referral needs to be taken into consideration. If the clinician is inquiring whether a generalized slow-wave abnormality exists in the EEG (i.e., ruling out a diffuse metabolic or degenerative process), an awake recording is sufficient. Neither the length of the recording nor the number of recording channels (8–10 channels are sufficient) is crucial, because such abnormalities tend to be readily apparent. The most important caveat is to make absolutely sure that the subject is fully awake (not drowsy) during the procedure. Such reassurance should be made explicit in the electroencephalographic report. In borderline cases the inclusion of at least 3 minutes of hyperventilation could further enhance the abnormality. If the slow-wave abnormality predicted is of a focal nature (e.g., following head injury), a longer recording (approximately 20 minutes) may be needed. In addition, the use of more recording electrodes allows for better localization of the abnormality. A 16-channel recording is usually sufficient for standard EEGs. Again, in borderline cases hyperventilation may further enhance the abnormality. If hyperventilation was performed the electroencephalographic report should clearly indicate whether (in the opinion of the electroencephalographic technologist) the hyperventilation effort was adequate and whether it produced any effect (either normal or pathological).

If, on the other hand, the referring clinician is interested in ruling out the possibility that epileptiform discharges exist in the EEG, a strictly awake EEG becomes woefully inadequate. In this situation, the inclusion of a sleep tracing (recording while patient is drowsy and asleep) becomes very important, because many types of paroxysmal discharge are activated by light sleep. Technicians should avoid recording deeper stages of sleep. The electroencephalographic report should clearly indicate whether or not sleep was attained (it is also better to specify the sleep stage during which recording was done). There are no studies that have examined the minimum duration of sleep to be considered adequate. The currently prevailing wisdom is that any length of sleep is adequate. It is also well known that serial recordings enhance the likelihood of finding abnormalities, particularly epileptiform abnormalities (Ajmone-Marsan and Zivin 1970). In our experience, the yield beyond two recordings does not justify the added expense. Because the stress of 24 hours of sleep deprivation may itself have activating properties for eliciting paroxysmal electroencephalographic discharges, it may be useful to obtain a second recording following sleep deprivation if the first EEG was normal.

When a specific area of involvement is suspected because of the patient's symptomatology, less commonly used electrode placements should be considered. Three uncommon placements have been well examined in epilepsy populations: true anterior temporal, sphenoidal, and nasopharyngeal electrodes. There are no studies that have specifically examined the usefulness of these electrode placements in neuropsychiatric populations. The nasopharyngeal electrodes are invasive and are accompanied by significant discomfort. More troublesome are the facts that they are often associated with pulse and respiration artifacts; they interfere with obtaining a sleep recording; and they often increase the irritability of the patient, which then leads to the generation of additional artifact. Their suitability in patients with mainly psychiatric symptoms is questionable (Struve and Feigenbaum 1981). On the other hand, the anterior temporal electrodes are completely noninvasive. Nonepileptiform abnormalities in patients over age 40 were enhanced by the use of these electrodes (Nowack et al. 1988). Sphenoidal electrodes were introduced by Jones (1951). Using a hollow needle, a fine electrode (insulated except at the tip) is inserted between the zygoma and the sigmoid notch in the mandible until it is in contact with the base of the skull lateral to the foramen ovale. Some studies of sphenoidal electrodes show an increase in abnormality in as many as 40.5% of seizure patients who had no other specific changes in waking or sleep EEGs (Kristensen and Sindrup 1978). Almost all clinical neurophysiology laboratories are familiar with these special electrode placements.

Evoked Potentials

Cerebral evoked potentials are a series of waves recordable at the surface (scalp) that result from brain stimulation (visual, auditory, somatosensory, and cognitive). These evoked potentials are usually of small magnitude compared with the ongoing electroencephalographic activity. When the stimuli are repeated and the recordings of electroencephalographic activity resulting from each stimulus are mathematically added together, the responses to the stimuli (which are by and large time-locked to the stimuli) will add up, whereas the ongoing electroencephalographic activity will cancel out. This procedure, called averaging, allows the small-magnitude evoked potentials to be visualized and examined. In special situations an evoked potential component may be seen with a single stimulus presentation. This is the exception to the rule.

When a stimulus is presented to the brain, it has to first travel through the receiving sensory organ and the brainstem (except for visual and olfactory stimuli) on its way to the primary cortical regions that mediate the particular sensory modality. In this discussion we focus on the auditory evoked responses. The early waves following an auditory stimulus are called the *brainstem auditory evoked responses.* These components reflect the intactness of the pathways they traverse and thus are of great interest to neurologists. On the other hand, these components are rarely abnormal in psychiatric conditions and are not easily influenced by psychological manipulations. They are therefore of lesser importance to behavioral researchers and to clinicians. After these early waves, a number of evoked-potential components can predictably be seen. These components are influenced by levels of arousal and attentional manipulations. They have been shown to be abnormal in many psychiatric conditions. Therefore they are of considerable interest to behavioral scientists and carry some promise that they may become useful clinically. Monte Buchsbaum (1977) labeled these components the *midlatency evoked responses* to differentiate them from the earlier brainstem auditory evoked responses and the later *event-related potentials* (ERPs). The three most examined midlatency components in the auditory modality are P50 (a positive component occurring between 35 and 80 msec after stimulus onset), N100 (a negative component occurring between 80 and 150 msec after stimulus onset), and P200 (a positive component occurring between 150 and 250 msec after stimulus onset). These components share the characteristic that their amplitude decreases with repetition (habituation or sensory gating).

The ERPs are by far the most challenging evoked potentials to record and are the most promising clinically. ERPs occur only in response to a psychological event. For example, the detection of a rare stimulus embedded within a group of more frequent stimuli will generate a P300 wave (a positive component occurring between 250 and 500 msec after stimulus onset). The P300 ERP is perhaps the most extensively examined evoked potential in psychiatry. Decreased amplitude of the P300 in schizophrenic patients has been documented in more than 100 publications over the last 30 years. Both amplitude and latency abnormalities of the P300 have been described in association with Alzheimer's disease. The P300 ERP was also found to be abnormal in a number of psychiatric conditions, thus creating difficulty in using it for differential diagnostic purposes. John Polich (1998) addressed these difficulties and pointed out the need for interlaboratory standardization of recording procedures. He suggested that the P300 may be useful as a general indicator of cognitive functioning.

Two other ERPs are worth mentioning here. The mismatch negativity is generated in a paradigm similar to the one eliciting the P300 except that subjects are usually attending to something other than the stimulus being presented. The mismatch negativity is considered to reflect preattentive information processing. Although the data are still relatively sparse, abnormalities of the mismatch negativity seem to be much more prevalent in schizophrenia than in other disorders that are frequently in the differential diagnosis, such as bipolar disorder. This differential prevalence of the abnormality makes this component a likely candidate for future clinical applications. Finally, the N400 (a negative component occurring around 400 msec after stimulus onset) is typically generated when a sentence ends with an anomalous word (e.g., "I played tennis with my *dog*"). This component may have clinical utility in probing learning disability, particularly that related to reading and comprehension.

Currently available data suggest that although evoked potentials may not be able to support a specific diagnosis, they can provide useful information regarding the information-processing capacity of a particular individual. Furthermore, suggestions about ways of bringing evoked-potential testing closer to full clinical utility are beginning to appear (Pratt 2000). Finally, given that the different evoked-potential components may be reflecting entirely different aspects of information processing, it has been suggested that batteries of evoked potentials or combination of evoked potential studies with other electrophysiological tests may yield better differential diagnostic capabilities. This remains to be seen through future studies.

Topographic Quantitative Electroencephalography

Quantitative electroencephalography is rapidly emerging as a powerful analytical process for evaluating electroencephalographic information (Hughes and John 1999; John and Prichep 1993; Prichep and John 1992). The process begins with the recording of a routine standard EEG as described above. After visual inspection to remove artifacts, artifact-free tracings of 2–3 minutes of eyes-closed waking EEG are subjected to analysis using the fast Fourier transform to quantify the power at each frequency of the EEG averaged across the entire sample. When the standard EEG is quantified in this fashion, information about the shape of waveforms is lost; because of this the method is not useful for detecting paroxysmal electroencephalographic abnormalities, for which recognition of waveform morphology is crucial. Quantification may have certain advantages for objectively defining the degree to which frequency and amplitude characteristics of the background electroencephalography deviate from normative population means. Despite the considerable promise of quantitative electroencephalography as a diagnostic tool for neuropsychiatric disorders, large-scale multicenter studies designed to demonstrate the clinical utility of these findings in specific clinical situations—particularly in comparison to unaided clinical judgments—have yet to appear in the literature.

When quantitative EEGs are performed in research settings (even for clinical purposes), the standards employed are very strict but may be colored by the particular expertise in the laboratory. Standards for evoked potentials, quantitative electroencephalography, and other electrophysiological testing in general clinical neurophysiology laboratories have been published. These standards are not specific and do not take into account the special needs and problems posed by psychiatric patients. Nonetheless, interpretation of quantitative electroencephalography (similar to interpretation of standard electroencephalography or evoked potentials) requires considerable skill and particularly knowledge of and ability to differentiate between activity of cerebral origin and activity of noncerebral origin (artifacts).

Polysomnography

As defined by the American Academy of Sleep Medicine (2000), polysomnography is the continuous and simultaneous recording of multiple physiological variables during sleep. These recordings can include an EEG, electro-oculogram, mental/submental (chin) electromyogram (these three variables are used to identify the different stages of sleep), and electrocardiogram; respiratory air flow and respiratory movements are recorded when sleep apnea is a likely contributor to the clinical picture. Recording of leg movements helps identify patients with an abnormal increase in periodic leg movement during sleep, a finding that has been reported in association with posttraumatic stress disorder (Ross et al. 1994). When sleep-related breathing disorders are suspected of contributing to the clinical presentation, polysomnographic evaluation remains the gold standard in the workup of such patients.

The majority of psychiatric disorders are accompanied by subjective and objective disturbances of sleep. For the most part, however, the findings are relatively nonspecific, and the cost of studies remains too high for routine clinical diagnostic or prognostic use. Sleep studies are likely to become clinically useful in the foreseeable future in the workup of mood disorders. A number of review articles have outlined the abnormalities in sleep architecture that are frequently associated with mood disorders. The sensitivity and specificity of abnormalities in electroencephalographic sleep measures as markers of depression vary according to the criteria values used, the statistical analysis utilized, and the reference groups included (Buysse and Kupfer 1990). This same group of investigators was able to develop a discriminant index score based on reduced latency of rapid eye movement (REM) onset, increased REM density, and decreased sleep efficiency (Thase et al. 1997). This index was reported to reliably discriminate between depressed patients (both inpatients and outpatients) and nondepressed control subjects. The bulk of the literature suggests that sleep abnormalities may be capable of providing some insight into differentiating between patients with pure depression and those with contributory Axis II disorders on the one hand and between those with depression with psychotic features and those with schizophrenia on the other hand. Large multicenter clinical trials are necessary to achieve such determinations.

In patients with schizophrenia, the presence of a narcoleptic syndrome should be suspected if hallucinations tend to occur more at sleep onset (hypnagogic) or on awakening (hypnopompic). Polysomnography can help with this particular differential diagnostic question. Although this situation is admittedly rare (Douglass et al. 1991), the differentiation is crucial because the treatment of the two conditions is dramatically different. It should be noted that the relatively high cost of sleep studies plays a significant role in limiting a wider utilization of examining sleep abnormalities in neuropsychiatric disorders.

Interpretation of sleep studies in psychiatric populations requires considerable knowledge of sleep recording technology, sleep disorders, psychiatric disorders, and all the possible environmental factors that are likely to affect the sleep architecture of an individual subject.

Electrophysiological Assessment Considerations for Selected Clinical Presentations

Habitual or Repeated Impulsive or Aggressive Behavior

The general category of habitual or repeated impulsive or aggressive behavior includes impulse dyscontrol syndrome, personality disorders (antisocial and borderline), frontal or temporal lobe pathologies leading to weakening of control mechanisms, and some cases of subnormal cognitive or psychotic conditions. Figure 3–3 provides an example of a diffuse epileptiform EEG in an adolescent with uncontrolled temper outbursts.

Patients diagnosed with antisocial personality disorder frequently harbor organic brain pathology that can be assessed with help of the EEG along with other neuroevaluative tools. Convit et al. (1991) demonstrated that violence was very significantly related to the hemispheric asymmetry in the EEG for the frontotemporal regions. These researchers provided evidence that with increased levels of violence a greater level of delta power in the left compared with the right hemisphere can be found. Wong et al. (1994) retrospectively examined the EEGs and CT scans of 372 male patients in a maximum-security mental hospital while blind to the specific histories of the individual patients. The researchers reported that 20% of the EEGs (and 41% of CT scans) were abnormal in the most violent patients compared with 2.4% of the EEGs (and 6.7% of CT scans) in the least violent patients. The prevalence of abnormal EEGs in clinical populations of aggressive patients varies widely, from a low of 6.6% in patients with rage attacks and episodic violent behavior (Riley and Niedermeyer 1978) to as high as 53% in patients diagnosed with antisocial personality disorder (Harper et al. 1972).

Whether the appearance of an abnormal EEG predicts a favorable therapeutic response to anticonvulsant medications is

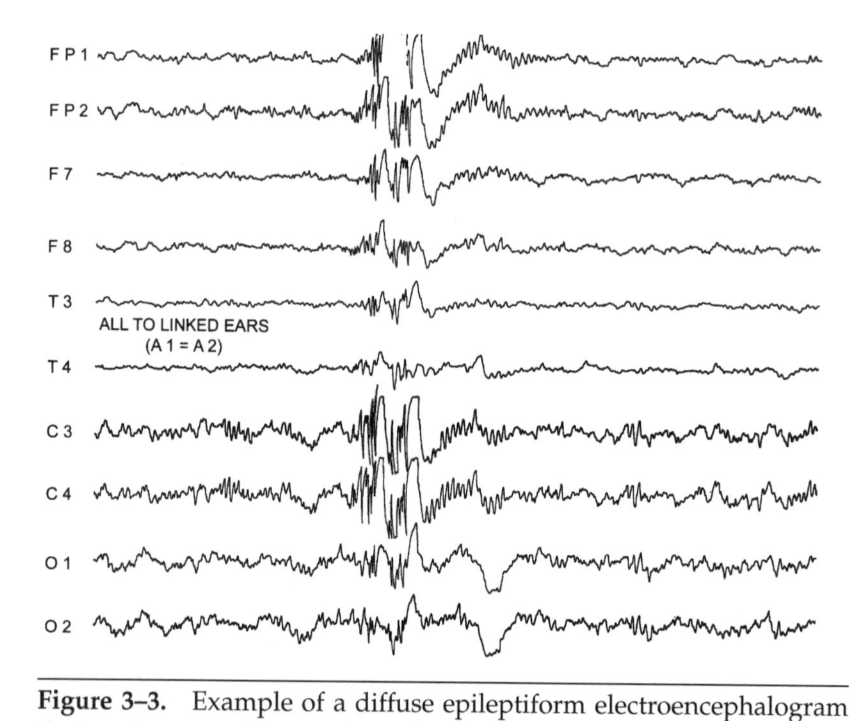

Figure 3–3. Example of a diffuse epileptiform electroencephalogram that can be seen with a variety of episodic behavioral symptoms.
Tracing is from a 15-year-old girl who was admitted for episodic confusion with serious temper dyscontrol as well as episodic dizzy spells.
Source. Reprinted from Boutros NN, Struve FA: "Applied Electrophysiology," in *Kaplan and Sadock's Comprehensive Textbook of Psychiatry,* 8th Edition. Edited by Sadock BJ, Sadock VA. Baltimore, MD, Lippincott Williams & Wilkins, in press. Used with permission.

currently unknown. Monroe (1975) showed that anticonvulsants can block electroencephalographic epileptiform discharges and can lead to dramatic clinical improvement in individuals exhibiting repeated and frequent aggressive behavior. Similarly, Neppe (1983) provided evidence that it can be clinically useful to add carbamazepine to the treatment of schizophrenic patients who also exhibit temporal lobe abnormalities on the EEG and who do not have a history of a seizure disorder. Earlier, Hakola and Laulumaa (1982) noted a reduction in aggressive episodes when carbamazepine was added to the neuroleptic regimen of eight highly aggressive women with schizophrenia who also had electroencephalographic abnormalities. On the other hand, other studies (Luchins 1984) suggest that anticonvulsant therapy may have a beneficial effect on aggressive tendencies irrespective of the presence or absence of electroencephalographic abnormalities. Until definitive studies are performed, patients should be given the benefit of the doubt and a trial of anticonvulsant should be performed when an EEG proves to be abnormal, particularly focally and paroxysmally.

Patients with a history of epilepsy or of episodic behavioral changes suggestive of epilepsy should have thorough neurological and electroencephalographic evaluations. The latter group includes patients with episodic dyscontrol (Monroe 1975) as well as patients who have dissociative disorders with features resembling complex partial seizures (Blumer et al. 1988; Mesulam 1981). A wide range of atypical labile pleomorphic psychiatric conditions respond well to carbamazepine. These disorders are characterized by evidence of central nervous system disturbance or family history of epilepsy and by mental changes typical of the interictal phase of temporal lobe epilepsy; in the absence of seizures they are identified as temporal lobe syndromes (Blumer et al. 1988).

Cognitive Decline

With early or mild cognitive decline the standard EEG is usually normal. However, the assessment of early cognitive decline may represent an area where topographic quantitative electroencephalographic methodology can make a strong clinical contribution (Prichep et al. 1994) both as an initial assessment and as a method of monitoring longitudinal change. This is because the quantification process can objectively identify small but statistically significant increases in slow-wave activity that would be difficult to reliably appreciate with visual inspection of the raw electroencephalographic tracing. There is a general agreement in the literature that increased slow-wave activity (initially in the theta range and later in the slower delta range) and decreased mean frequency are correlated with cognitive impairment and measures of clinical severity of Alzheimer's disease (Brenner et al. 1986; Robinson et al. 1994). Many workers regard increased slow-wave activity before reduction of alpha power as the earliest electrophysiological indicator of Alzheimer's disease (Coburn et al. 1985). Alzheimer's disease and multi-infarct dementia have been differentiated by evaluating asymmetry of slow-wave activity (Martin-Loeches et al. 1991). Similarly, quantitative electroencephalography can be helpful in differentiating Alzheimer's disease from frontotemporal dementia (Yener et al. 1996). It should be noted that the P300 cognitive evoked potential may also be of value with such patients (Polich and Herbst 2000).

Based on our evaluation of this literature, we conclude that quantitative electroencephalography or a battery of quantitative electroencephalography and ERP tests (P300) are ready for large-scale multicenter studies designed to characterize their usefulness in the actual clinical setting.

Advanced Dementia

Although the clinical picture is usually clear when dementia is in an advanced stage, issues of differential diagnosis sometimes arise. Particularly problematic is the question of depression or pseudodementia. Patients with advanced dementia rarely have a normal EEG (Hooner et al. 1990). For this reason, a normal standard EEG can play an important role in diagnosing cases of pseudodementia. When dementia and depression coexist, it becomes important to have some idea about the relative contribution of each disorder to the overall clinical presentation. In this respect it has been shown (Brenner et al. 1989) that when comparisons were made between the EEGs of patients with depression, dementia, pseudodementia, and dementia plus depression and the EEGs of healthy age-matched control subjects, the degree of electroencephalographic abnormality showed a significant inverse association with clinical response to antidepressants. Multiple studies report accurate discrimination of Alzheimer's disease patients from depressed patients by use of both standard and quantitative electroencephalography (Brenner et al. 1986; Robinson et al. 1994). The P300 ERP and sleep studies examining this differential diagnostic issue are also potentially useful. Larger-scale studies defining the utility of these tests individually or in test batteries have yet to be reported.

Acute Confusion or Disorganization

The differential diagnosis of acutely disturbed and disorganized psychotic patients often includes delirium. In acutely agitated patients with delirium, the EEG is often helpful in indicating whether the alteration in consciousness is due to 1) a diffuse encephalopathic process, 2) a focal brain lesion (see Figure 3–4), or 3) continued epileptic activity without motor manifestations. Most often, patients with delirium have a toxic-metabolic encephalopathy. In general, with the progression of the encephalopathy there is diffuse slowing of the background rhythms from alpha (8–13 Hz) to theta (4–7.5 Hz) activity. Delta (<3.5 Hz) activity usually does not become prominent until the patient approaches nonresponsiveness. The major exception to this rule is seen during withdrawal from alcohol and during delirium tremens. Excessive fast activity (rather than slowing) dominates the EEG in patients with alcohol withdrawal delirium, whereas patients in alcohol withdrawal who are not delirious could have a normal EEG (Reilly et al. 1979). It should be noted that low-voltage fast activity is almost always induced by benzodiazepines; clinicians should bear this in mind when interpreting EEGs. For a review of the role of electroencephalography in diagnosing and managing delirium, with emphasis on the elderly, the interested reader is referred to Brenner (1991). It should be pointed out that obtaining adequate recordings from agitated and uncooperative patients is technically very challenging. The availability of electroencephalographic technicians with significant expertise in working with psychotic, manic, or agitated patients is essential. Moreover, proficiency in the use of electrode caps can facilitate the process by decreasing the time necessary for applying scalp electrodes.

Attentional Problems

Core attentional disorders may need to be separated from a variety of differential diagnoses, including bipolar disorder, learning disability, certain personality disorders, behavioral problems, and epileptic disorders. There is a steadily increasing body of literature describing electroencephalographic frequency changes (par-

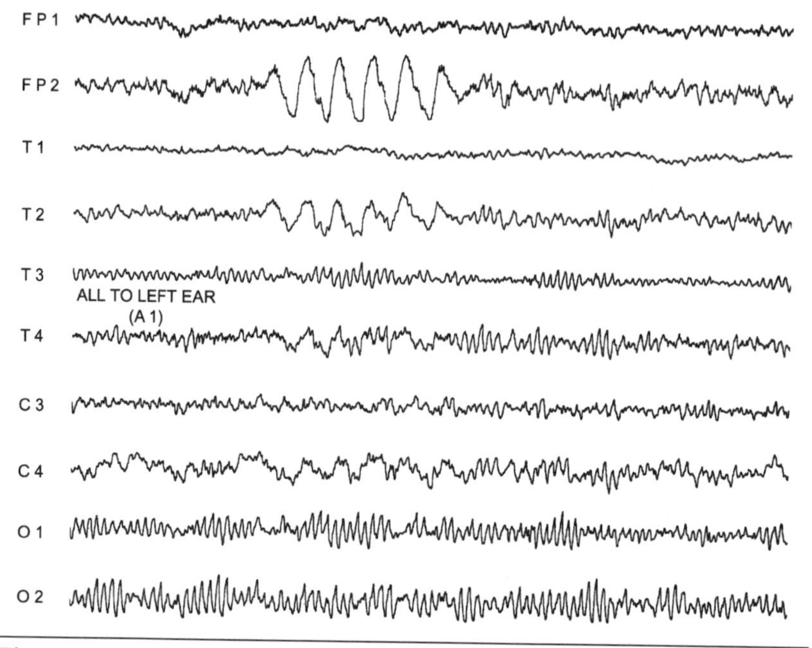

Figure 3–4. Example of a focal electroencephalographic abnormality associated with episodic confusion.
Focal slow-wave (delta) activity in the right prefrontal cortex spreading to the right anterior temporal–midtemporal–central cortex. Tracing is from a previously well-functioning 49-year-old professional woman with no prior psychiatric history. Beginning 6 months before the electroencephalogram she began to display increasing periods of episodic confusion.
Source. Reprinted from Boutros NN, Struve FA: "Applied Electrophysiology," in *Kaplan and Sadock's Comprehensive Textbook of Psychiatry,* 8th Edition. Edited by Sadock BJ, Sadock VA. Baltimore, MD, Lippincott Williams & Wilkins, in press. Used with permission.

ticularly increased theta waves) among patients with attention-deficit/hyperactivity disorder (ADHD), and evidence shows that the degree of electroencephalographic alteration may be related to academic performance (Harmony et al. 1990). Although these electroencephalographic findings may assist in the differentiation between genuine attentional disorders and other behavioral problems associated with a normal EEG, the findings are still not specific to attentional deficits or learning disabilities, and their clinical diagnostic significance remains uncertain. The incidence of positive electroencephalographic findings is also increased in personality disorders. However, here the array of findings is highly variable with no specific electroencephalographic correlates to these disorders (Hughes 1995). In contrast to pure attentional disorders, personality disorders are often more likely to display epileptiform or controversial paroxysmal findings, particularly if aggressive acting out is part of the symptom complex (Boutros and Struve 2002).

Frank (1993) reported that 36% (25 of 68) of a sample of 7- to 12-year-old children diagnosed with ADHD had abnormal routine EEGs. Of the 25 children with abnormal EEGs, 21 (84%) had spikes or spike-wave discharges. The others had slowing of the background in excess of what was expected for age. In 1998, Boutros et al. reported an association between ADHD and the 14- and 6-per-second positive spikes in children and adolescents. This electroencephalographic pattern is controversial but has been linked to a variety of behavioral abnormalities, including episodic somatic symptoms and hyperactivity, and emotional instability. More recently, Wojna et al. (2000) further confirmed that approximately one-third of children with ADHD had an abnormal routine EEG, with a sizable proportion exhibiting epileptiform activity. The same result was reported by Gustafsson et al. (2000), when they found that 10 of 28 (36%) children with ADHD had electroencephalographic abnormalities. Finally, Hemmer et al. (2001) reported that of 234 children (179 boys age 9.1 ± 3.6 years and 55 girls age 9.6 ± 3.9 years), 36 (15.4%) had epileptiform abnormalities. These researchers did not include any of the controversial electroencephalographic waveforms such as the 14- and 6-per-second positive spikes, thus explaining (at least in part) the lower rate of abnormalities in their sample. They further reported that methylphenidate therapy increased the risk for seizures, with an incidence of 0.6% in subjects with normal EEGs and 10% in subjects with epileptiform EEGs before administration of methylphenidate.

Increased theta activity, particularly in the frontal lobe regions, in children with attention-deficit disorder or ADHD has been reported by a number of independent research groups. This is a quantitative electroencephalographic finding. Lubar (1991) reviewed the then-existing literature regarding spectral electroencephalographic and evoked-potential abnormalities reported in association with ADHD. He listed excessive theta activity as the most consistent finding in this group. This group of researchers have investigated this problem for a considerable period of time. In 1990 the same group examined ADHD patients without a confounding learning disability (Mann et al. 1992) and reported the same finding of increased theta activity, mainly in the frontotemporal regions. Defrance et al. (1996) confirmed the increased theta activity, but they were unable to point out a specific neuroanatomical locus for the abnormality in their patient population. Lazzaro et al. (1998, 1999) further independently confirmed the finding in 26 male patients with combined ADHD and later in 54 similarly diagnosed subjects. (It is not clear whether subjects in the earlier study were part of the sample reported in the later study.) These researchers found the abnormality to be maximally seen in the anterior cerebral regions. In another independent replication study, Bresnahan et al. (1999) examined the age effects on the reported spectral electroencephalographic abnormalities. They concluded that the theta excess is consistent and is resistant to age effects, whereas beta abnormalities tended to decrease with age. Most recently, Clarke et al. (2001a) further confirmed the abnormality in a group of 40 boys and 40 girls. These researchers suggested that the theta-to-beta ratio provides a stronger measure of the abnormality. This ratio measure combines the abnormalities of the theta rhythm with abnormalities in beta activity (usually a decrease in beta activity that is less consistently reported) for a higher detection power. The researchers nevertheless showed that the theta excess was statistically demonstrable without using the ratio measure (using absolute theta power) (Clarke et al. 2001b), which further confirmed their earlier similar finding (Clarke et al. 1998).

Ucles and Lorente (1996) found the increase in theta activity to be more prominent in the occipital region of a similar group of subjects. In this study the researchers used a theta-alpha index to compare groups. They also found the theta-alpha index to be borderline abnormal in the frontal regions. It should be noted that in two studies an increase (rather than a decrease) in beta activity was found in similar groups of patients (Clarke et al. 2001c;

Kuperman et al. 1996). A distinct subgroup of ADHD patients with increased beta activity may exist, but this conclusion awaits replication of the finding and identification of the clinical correlates of this subgroup. Lazzaro et al. (2001) reported the same finding and suggested that the combination of electroencephalographic and ERP examinations may be more powerful than either examination alone. Finally, Kovatchev et al. (2001) proposed that an electroencephalographic consistency index derived from the same data may further add to the diagnostic ability of the EEG.

Evoked potential abnormalities (P300) have also been reported in association with attention-deficit disorder and ADHD. As early as the Lubar review (1991) it was obvious that a number of evoked potential abnormalities are detectable in association with ADHD. These include a decrease in the amplitude of the P300, N100, and P200 components. These abnormalities have also been replicated, suggesting that electrophysiological abnormalities are somewhat prevalent in this group of patients. In particular, the P300 component has repeatedly been shown to be deficient in amplitude in children with ADHD. Additional abnormalities were identified for the N200 and the negative difference component of the mismatch negativity (Satterfield et al. 1988). A rather limited body of literature involves attempts to combine electroencephalographic and ERP measures to delineate the clinical usefulness of each of the modalities, but attempts at combining the tests in the form of a battery to examine improvement in diagnostic sensitivity and specificity were not done.

In summary, the available literature appears to suggest that in cases of severe ADHD—especially if epileptic activity such as petit mal or temporal lobe epilepsy is suspected—a standard EEG should be obtained. It is our assessment that the quantitative electroencephalographic finding of increased theta activity or increased theta activity relative to beta activity has been replicated enough to be considered a highly promising candidate for a diagnostic test for ADHD. Multicenter studies designed to define the clinical utility of quantitative electroencephalography or a battery of quantitative electroencephalographic and ERP tests should help accomplish this goal.

Rapid-Cycling Bipolar Disorder

Patients with rapid-cycling bipolar disorder may exhibit epileptiform discharges on their EEG. More than a decade ago, Levy and associates (1988) reported that three of five patients with rapid cycling had paroxysmal sharp wave discharges in their EEGs, whereas none of a comparison sample of 25 patients with non–rapid-cycling bipolar disorder displayed such electroencephalographic findings. This finding may explain the reported efficacy of anticonvulsants for rapid-cycling bipolar disorders. Others (Himmelhoch 1987) have recognized a variety of clinical characteristics in some bipolar patients—including episodic hostile outbursts, sudden plunges into depression marked by impulsive suicidal behavior, hyperirritability, sudden euphoric periods, and compulsive symptoms—that combined may constitute a subictal mood disorder. Both frank paroxysmal electroencephalographic epileptiform discharges and controversial paroxysmal waveforms would be expected with such symptom complexes. Patients with subictal mood disorders may also have paradoxical reactions to mood-active drugs (lithium and antidepressants), with better response to anticonvulsants.

Panic Attacks

Panic symptoms carry a significant resemblance to symptoms induced by temporolimbic epileptic activity, particularly those originating from the Sylvian fissure. Fear, derealization, tachycardia, diaphoresis, and abdominal discomfort are characteristic symptoms of simple partial seizures with psychiatric and autonomic symptomatology. Evidence from population surveys suggests that panic disorder is significantly more prevalent in epileptic patients than in the general public (Pariente et al. 1991). Toni et al. (1996) compared the symptoms of 91 patients with panic disorder and agoraphobia and 41 patients with complex partial epileptic seizures. The researchers found many similarities and concluded that there may be a common neurophysiological substrate linking complex partial seizures and panic disorder with agoraphobia. A number of reports provide evidence that electroencephalographic abnormalities are not infrequent in patients with panic disorder. Weilburg et al. (1995) reported on 15 subjects with atypical panic attacks who met DSM-III-R criteria for panic disorder (American Psychiatric Association 1987) and who underwent a routine EEG followed by prolonged ambulatory electroencephalographic monitoring using sphenoidal electrodes. The researchers found focal paroxysmal electroencephalographic changes consistent with partial seizure activity that occurred during a panic attack in 5 (33%) of the subjects. It is important to note that multiple attacks were recorded before panic-related electroencephalographic changes were demonstrated. Moreover, 2 of the 5 subjects with demonstrated electroencephalographic abnormalities during panic attacks had perfectly normal baseline EEGs. The researchers concluded that it may be necessary to monitor the EEG during multiple attacks to reveal an association between atypical panic attacks and epileptiform electroencephalographic changes. Polysomnography can be quite useful in differentiating nocturnal nonepileptic attacks from epileptic seizures (Roberts 1998).

Finally, computerized electroencephalography promises to provide further refinement to the utility of electroencephalography in detecting abnormalities in patients with panic disorder and to the overall diagnostic accuracy of electroencephalography. Abraham and Duffy (1991) were able to differentiate between patients with panic disorder and control subjects with 92.5% accuracy.

Conclusion and Recommendations

At the current time the potential clinical usefulness of neuropsychiatric electrophysiology remains largely unappreciated. This is evidenced by the fact that psychiatry residents are not exposed to electrophysiology in any systematized or organized fashion. Indeed, the number of academic psychiatric departments that provide clinical electrophysiology testing can be counted on one hand. This is unfortunate, because the standard EEG constitutes a testing modality with several well-established clinical applications. Other electrophysiological measures that are potentially clinically useful include quantified electroencephalography, cerebral evoked potentials, and polysomnography. Although magnetoencephalography is an important research investigative tool that ultimately may have considerable clinical promise, its usefulness in routine clinical psychiatry is hampered at present due to the cost associated with setting up the apparatus and the need for expensive maintenance and specialized knowledge in running and maintaining the equipment.

An added level of complexity for neurobehavioral electrophysiology is the sensitivity of the measures to psychological factors such as attention for event-related potentials and the first-night effect for sleep studies. At present there are no clinical behavioral electrophysiology training programs that will guarantee a comprehensive exposure to all electrophysiological modalities. Likewise, there are no certifying organizations similar to the American Board of Clinical Neurophysiology and no additional qualifications (such as that in clinical neurophysiology administered by the American Board of Psychiatry and Neurology) that are specifically designed to ensure competence in behavioral or neuropsychiatric electrophysiology.

The rapid evolution of the American Neuropsychiatric Association is a major and significant advance toward the goal of establishing a neuropsychiatric discipline similar to the discipline of clinical neurophysiology but with a focus on behavioral electrophysiology. The second major advance is the establishment of the EEG and Clinical Neuroscience Society. The EEG and Clinical Neuroscience Society is the first independent scientific organization whose main purpose is to disseminate knowledge regarding the electrophysiology of neuropsychiatric disorders, encourage translational research to bring the many scientific discoveries in neuropsychiatric electrophysiology to bear on the clinical practice of this field, as well as organizing and leading the development of the clinical discipline itself.

Although electrophysiological testing continues to play a marginal role in the diagnosis and management of neuropsychiatric disorders, it seems that currently available knowledge should allow better utilization of these resources. Moreover, the evidence suggests that progressively more clinical applications are likely to become accepted as the sensitivities and specificities of abnormalities are better defined and as standardization of methodology is undertaken. Future studies with a focus on defining the clinical utility of these modalities should be designed with patient control groups that are specifically relevant to the differential diagnostic process and with adequate attention to the issue of the gold standard for diagnosis. In fact, studies reporting on the clinical applications of laboratory tests should adhere to the criteria specified in the Standard for Reporting Diagnostic Tests (Bossuyt et al. 2003; Bruns 2003). Adherence to such standards is crucial, because evidence of design-related bias in studies of diagnostic tests has been reported (Lijmer et al. 1999). Interested researchers are referred to a body of work by Somoza and his co-workers (see Somoza and Kim 1999 for an overview).

Finally, we believe that the development of specialized fellowship training programs for clinical electrophysiology within the field of psychiatry will help create a generation of psychiatrists and psychologists who are skilled both clinically and electrophysiologically. Currently available research fellowships tend to focus on research questions and rarely expose the trainee to more than a single testing modality.

References

Abraham HD, Duffy FH: Computed EEG abnormalities in panic disorder with and without premorbid drug abuse. Biol Psychiatry 29:687–690, 1991

Ajmone-Marsan C, Zivin LS: Factors related to the occurrence of typical paroxysmal abnormalities in the EEG records of epileptic patients. Epilepsia 11:361–381, 1970

American Academy of Sleep Medicine: The International Classification of Sleep Disorders. Revised: Diagnostic and Coding Manual. Rochester, MN, American Academy of Sleep Medicine, 2000

American Psychiatric Association: Diagnostic and Statistical Manual of Mental Disorders, 3rd Edition, Revised. Washington, DC, American Psychiatric Association, 1987

American Psychiatric Association: Diagnostic and Statistical Manual of Mental Disorders, 4th Edition. Washington, DC, American Psychiatric Association, 1994

American Psychiatric Association: Diagnostic and Statistical Manual of Mental Disorders, 4th Edition, Text Revision. Washington, DC, American Psychiatric Association, 2000

Blumer D, Heilbronn M, Himmelhoch J: Indications for carbamazepine in mental illness: atypical psychiatric disorder or temporal lobe syndrome? Compr Psychiatry 29:108–122, 1988

Bossuyt PM, Reitsma JB, Bruns DE, et al: Towards complete and accurate reporting of studies of diagnostic accuracy: the STARD initiative. Clin Chem 49:1–6, 2003

Boutros NN, Struve FA: Electrophysiological assessment of neuropsychiatric disorders. Semin Clin Neuropsychiatry 7:30–41, 2002

Boutros N, Fristad M, Abdollohian A: The fourteen and six positive spikes and attention-deficit hyperactivity disorder. Biol Psychiatry 44:298–301, 1998

Brenner RP: Utility of electroencephalography in delirium: past views and current practice. Int Psychogeriatr 3:211–229, 1991

Brenner RP, Ulrich RF, Spiker DG: Computerized EEG spectral analysis in elderly normal, demented and depressed subjects. Electroencephalogr Clin Neurophysiol 64:483–492, 1986

Brenner RP, Reynolds CF, Ulrich RF: EEG findings in depressive pseudodementia and dementia with secondary depression. Electroencephalogr Clin Neurophysiol 72:293–304, 1989

Bresnahan SM, Anderson JW, Barry RJ: Age-related changes in quantitative EEG in attention-deficit/hyperactivity disorder. Biol Psychiatry 46:1690–1697, 1999

Bruns DE: The STARD initiative and the reporting of studies of diagnostic accuracy. Clin Chem 49:19–20, 2003

Buchsbaum MS: The middle evoked response components and schizophrenia. Schizophr Bull 3:93–104, 1977

Buysse DJ, Kupfer DJ: Diagnostic and research applications of electroencephalographic sleep studies in depression: conceptual and methodological issues. J Nerv Ment Dis 178:404–414, 1990

Clarke AR, Barry RJ, McCarthy R, et al: EEG analysis in attention-deficit/hyperactivity disorder: a comparative study of two subtypes. Psychiatry Res 81:19–29, 1998

Clarke AR, Barry RJ, McCarthy R, et al: Age and sex effects in the EEG: differences in two subtypes of attention-deficit/hyperactivity disorder. Clin Neurophysiol 112:815–826, 2001a

Clarke AR, Barry RJ, McCarthy R, et al: Electroencephalogram differences in two subtypes of attention-deficit/hyperactivity disorder. Psychophysiology 38:212–221, 2001b

Clarke AR, Barry RJ, McCarthy R, et al: Excess beta activity in children with attention-deficit/hyperactivity disorder: an atypical electrophysiological group. Psychiatry Res 103:205–218, 2001c

Coburn KA, Danziger WL, Storandt M: A longitudinal EEG study of mild senile dementia of Alzheimer's type: changes at 1 year and at 2.5 years. Electroencephalogr Clin Neurophysiol 61:101–112, 1985

Convit A, Czobor P, Volavka J: Lateralized abnormality in the EEG of persistently violent psychiatric inpatients. Biol Psychiatry 30:363–370, 1991

Defrance JF, Smith S, Schweitzer FC, et al: Topographical analysis of attention disorders of childhood. Int J Neurosci 87:41–61, 1996

Douglass AB, Hays P, Pazderka F, et al: Florid refractory schizophrenias that turn out to be treatable variants of HLA-associated narcolepsy. J Nerv Ment Dis 179:12–17, 1991

Feinstein AR: Clinical Biostatistics. St. Louis, MO, CV Mosby, 1977

Frank Y: Visual event related potentials after methylphenidate and sodium valproate in children with attention deficit hyperactivity disorder. Clin Electroencephalogr 24:19–24, 1993

Gustafsson P, Thernlund G, Ryding E: Associations between cerebral blood-flow measured by single photon emission computed tomography (SPECT), electro-encephalogram (EEG), behaviour symptoms, cognitive and neurological soft signs in children with attention-deficit hyperactivity disorder (ADHD). Acta Paediatr 89:830–835, 2000

Hakola HP, Laulumaa VA: Carbamazepine in treatment of violent schizophrenics (letter). Lancet 1:1358, 1982

Harmony T, Hinojosa G, Marosi E, et al: Correlation between EEG spectral parameters and an educational evaluation. Int J Neurosci 54:147–155, 1990

Harper MA, Morris M, Bleyerveld J: The significance of an abnormal EEG in psychopathic personalities. Aust N Z J Psychiatry 6:215–224, 1972

Hemmer SA, Pasternak JF, Zecker SG, et al: Stimulant therapy and seizure risk in children with ADHD. Pediatr Neurol 24:99–102, 2001

Himmelhoch JM: Cerebral dysrhythmia, substance abuse, and the nature of secondary affective illness. Psychiatr Ann 17:710–727, 1987

Hooner C, Jonker C, Posthuma J: Reliability, validity, and follow-up of the EEG in senile dementia: sequential measurements. Electroencephalogr Clin Neurophysiol 76:400–412, 1990

Hughes JR: The EEG in psychiatry: an outline with summarized points and references. Clin Electroencephalogr 26:92–101, 1995

Hughes JR, Gruener G: Small sharp spikes revisited: further data on this controversial pattern. Clin Electroencephalogr 15:208–213, 1984

Hughes JR, John ER: Conventional and quantitative electroencephalography in psychiatry. J Neuropsychiatry Clin Neurosci 11:190–208, 1999

Inui K, Mtomura E, Okushima R, et al: Electroencephalographic findings in patients with DSM-IV mood disorder, schizophrenia and other psychotic disorders. Biol Psychiatry 43:69–75, 1998

John ER, Prichep LS: Principles of neurometrics and neurometric analysis of EEG and evoked potentials, in Electroencephalography: Basic Principles, Clinical Applications and Related Fields. Edited by Niedermeyer E, Lopes da Silva F. Baltimore, MD, Williams & Wilkins, 1993, pp 989–1003

Jones DP: Recording on the basal electroencephalogram with sphenoidal needle electrodes (abstract). Electroencephalogr Clin Neurophysiol 3:100, 1951

Kovatchev B, Cox D, Hill R, et al: A psychophysiological marker of attention deficit/hyperactivity disorder (ADHD)—defining the EEG consistency index. Appl Psychophysiol Biofeedback 26:127–139, 2001

Kristensen O, Sindrup EH: Psychomotor epilepsy and psychosis, II: electroencephalographic findings (sphenoidal electrode recordings). Acta Neurol Scand 57:370–379, 1978

Kuperman S, Johnson B, Arndt S, et al: Quantitative EEG differences in a nonclinical sample of children with ADHD and undifferentiated ADD. J Am Acad Child Adolesc Psychiatry 35:1009–1017, 1996

Lazzaro I, Gordon E, Whitmont S, et al: Quantified EEG activity in adolescent attention deficit hyperactivity disorder. Clin Electroencephalogr 29:37–42, 1998

Lazzaro I, Gordon E, Li W, et al: Simultaneous EEG and EDA measures in adolescent attention deficit hyperactivity disorder. Int J Psychophysiol 34:123–134, 1999

Lazzaro I, Gordon E, Whitmont S, et al: The modulation of late component event related potentials by pre-stimulus EEG theta activity in ADHD. Int J Neurosci 107:247–264, 2001

Leckman JF, Sholomskas D, Thompson WD, et al: Best estimate of lifetime psychiatric diagnosis: a methodological study. Arch Gen Psychiatry 39:879–883, 1982

Levy AB, Drake ME, Shy KE: EEG evidence of epileptiform paroxysms in rapid cycling bipolar patients. J Clin Psychiatry 49:232–234, 1988

Lijmer JG, Mol BW, Heisterkamp S, et al: Empirical evidence of design-related bias in studies of diagnostic tests. JAMA 282:1061–1066, 1999

Lubar JF: Discourse on the development of EEG diagnostics and biofeedback for attention-deficit/hyperactivity disorders. Biofeedback Self Regul 16:201–225, 1991

Luchins DJ: Carbamazepine in violent non-epileptic schizophrenics. Psychopharmacol Bull 20:569–571, 1984

Mann CA, Lubar JF, Zimmerman AW, et al: Quantitative analysis of EEG in boys with attention-deficit-hyperactivity disorder: controlled study with clinical implications. Pediatr Neurol 8:30–36, 1992

Martin-Loeches M, Gil P, Jimenez F, et al: Topographic maps of brain electrical activity in primary degenerative dementia of Alzheimer type and multi-infarct dementia. Biol Psychiatry 29:211–223, 1991

Mesulam MM: Dissociative states with abnormal temporal lobe EEG. Arch Neurol 38:176–181, 1981

Monroe RR: Anticonvulsants in the treatment of aggression. J Nerv Ment Dis 160:119–126, 1975

Neppe VM: Carbamazepine as adjunctive treatment in nonepileptic chronic inpatients with EEG temporal lobe abnormalities. J Clin Psychiatry 44:326–331, 1983

Nowack WJ, Janati A, Metzer WS, et al: The anterior temporal electrodes in the EEG of the adult. Clin Electroencephalogr 19:199–204, 1988

Nuwer M: Uses and abuses of brain mapping. Arch Neurol 46:1134–1136, 1989

Pariente PD, Lepine JP, Lellouch J: Lifetime history of panic attacks and epilepsy: an association from a general population survey. J Clin Psychiatry 52:88–89, 1991

Polich J: P300 clinical utility and control of variability. J Clin Neurophysiol 15:14–33, 1998

Polich J, Herbst KL: P300 as a clinical assay: rationale, evaluation, and findings. Int J Psychophysiol 38:3–19, 2000

Pratt H: Improving the clinical utility of event-related potentials. Clin Neurophysiol 111:1425–1426, 2000

Prichep LS, John ER: QEEG profiles of psychiatric disorders. Brain Topogr 4:249–257, 1992

Prichep LS, John ER, Ferris SH, et al: Quantitative EEG correlates of cognitive deterioration in the elderly. Neurobiol Aging 15:85–90, 1994

Reilly EL, Glass G, Faillace LA: EEGs in an alcohol detoxification and treatment center. Clin Electroencephalogr 10:69–71, 1979

Riley T, Niedermeyer E: Rage attacks and episodic violent behavior: electroencephalographic findings and general considerations. Clin Electroencephalogr 9:131–139, 1978

Roberts R: Differential diagnosis of sleep disorders, nonepileptic attacks and epileptic seizures. Curr Opin Neurol 11:135–139, 1998

Robinson DJ, Merskey H, Blume WT, et al: Electroencephalography as an aid in the exclusion of Alzheimer's disease. Arch Neurol 51:280–284, 1994

Ross RJ, Ball WA, Dinges DF, et al: Motor dysfunction during sleep in posttraumatic stress disorder. Sleep 17:723–732, 1994

Roy MA, Lanctot G, Merette C, et al: Clinical and methodological factors related to reliability of the best-estimate diagnostic procedure. Am J Psychiatry 154:1726–1733, 1997

Saito F, Fukushima Y, Kubota S: Small sharp spikes: possible relationship to epilepsy. Clin Electroencephalogr 18:114–119, 1987

Satterfield JH, Schell AM, Nicholas T, et al: Topographic study of auditory event-related potentials in normal boys and boys with attention deficit with hyperactivity. Psychophysiology 25:591–606, 1988

Somoza E, Kim S: What would it take for electrophysiology to become clinically useful? CNS Spectr 4(8):1–8, 1999

Steffens DC, Krishnan KRR: Laboratory testing and neuroimaging, in Advancing DSM: Dilemmas in Psychiatric Diagnosis. Edited by Philips KA, First MB, Pincus HA. Washington, DC, American Psychiatric Association, 2003, pp 85–103

Struve FA: Clinical electroencephalography as an assessment method in psychiatric practice, in Handbook of Psychiatric Diagnostic Procedures. Edited by Hall RC, Beresford T. New York, Spectrum, 1985, pp 1–48

Struve FA, Feigenbaum ZS: Experience with nasopharyngeal electrode recording with psychiatric patients: a clinical note. Clin Electroencephalogr 12:84–88, 1981

Thase ME, Kupfer DJ, Fasiczka AJ, et al: Identifying an abnormal electroencephalographic sleep profile to characterize major depressive disorder. Biol Psychiatry 41:964–973, 1997

Toni C, Cassano GB, Perugi G, et al: Psychosensorial and related phenomena in panic disorder and in temporal lobe epilepsy. Compr Psychiatry 37:125–133, 1996

Ucles P, Lorente S: Electrophysiologic measures of delayed maturation in attention-deficit hyperactivity disorder. J Child Neurol 11:155–156, 1996

Weilburg JB, Schachter S, Worth J, et al: EEG abnormalities in patients with atypical panic attacks. J Clin Psychiatry 56:358–362, 1995

Wojna V, Rosa J, Borras JV, et al: EEG in attention deficit disorder. Paper presented at the annual meeting of the American Clinical Neurophysiology Society, Montreal, Canada, September 2000
Wong MTH, Lumsden J, Fenton GW, et al: Electroencephalography, computed tomography and violence ratings of male patients in a maximum-security mental hospital. Acta Psychiatr Scand 90:97–101, 1994
Yener GG, Leuchter AF, Jenden D: Quantitative EEG in frontotemporal dementia. Clin Electroencephalogr 27:61–68, 1996

Chapter 4

Neuropsychiatric Laboratory Testing

H. Florence Kim, M.D.
Stuart C. Yudofsky, M.D.

Laboratory assessment is essential to the neuropsychiatric workup of the psychiatric patient. Neuropsychiatry is primarily focused on the assessment and treatment of the cognitive, behavioral, and mood symptoms of patients with neurological disorders, as well as the understanding of the role of brain dysfunction in primary psychiatric disorders. Laboratory assessment is particularly important to the neuropsychiatric approach because of the complex variety of neurological and medical illnesses that may underlie the psychiatric symptoms of a neuropsychiatric patient. A careful neuropsychiatric history and physical examination and judicious clinical laboratory testing can focus or even obviate neuroimaging or electrophysiological testing, which can be expensive, invasive, and physically and emotionally uncomfortable for the patient. Unlike primary mood and psychotic disorders, neuropsychiatric disorders often have clinical pathology that is evident through abnormalities in laboratory tests. Furthermore, psychiatric symptoms that on the surface may appear to be similar may in fact have dissimilar etiologies. For example, hallucinations can occur in the context of schizophrenia as well as in Alzheimer's disease, frontotemporal dementia, delirium from other chronic medical illnesses, and alcohol withdrawal. Table 4–1 lists some of the many medical and neurological illnesses that may present with prominent neuropsychiatric symptoms. Clinical laboratory assessment and diagnostic testing can help one determine which of these many underlying causes is responsible for a patient's hallucinations. Importantly, a number of these etiologies may have potentially curative remediations, as opposed to only symptomatic treatment.

Table 4–1. Selected medical conditions with neuropsychiatric manifestations

Neurological
Cerebrovascular disease
Multiple sclerosis
Multiple systems atrophy
Parkinson's disease
Progressive supranuclear palsy
Alzheimer's disease
Frontotemporal dementias
Dementia associated with Lewy bodies
Seizure disorder
Huntington's disease
Traumatic brain injury
Anoxic brain injury
Migraine headache
Sleep disorders (narcolepsy, sleep apnea)
Normal pressure hydrocephalus
Neoplastic
Central nervous system tumors, primary and metastatic
Pancreatic carcinoma
Paraneoplastic syndromes
Endocrine tumors
Pheochromocytoma
Infectious
Human immunodeficiency virus infection
Neurosyphilis
Creutzfeldt-Jacob disease
Systemic viral and bacterial infections
Viral and bacterial meningitis and encephalitis
Tuberculosis
Infectious mononucleosis
Pediatric autoimmune neuropsychiatric disorder associated with streptococcal infections

Table 4–1. Selected medical conditions with neuropsychiatric manifestations *(continued)*

Nutritional
Vitamin deficiencies
B_{12}: pernicious anemia
Folate: megaloblastic anemia
Nicotinic acid: pellagra
Thiamine: Wernicke-Korsakoff syndrome
Trace mineral deficiency (zinc, magnesium)
Autoimmune
Systemic lupus erythematosus
Sarcoidosis
Sjögren's syndrome
Behçet's syndrome
Endocrine/metabolic
Wilson's disease
Fluid and electrolyte disturbances: syndrome of inappropriate antidiuretic hormone secretion, central pontine myelinolysis
Porphyrias
Uremias
Hypercapnia
Hepatic encephalopathy
Hypercalcemia and hypocalcemia
Hyperglycemia and hypoglycemia
Thyroid and parathyroid disease
Diabetes mellitus
Pheochromocytoma
Pregnancy
Gonadotropic hormonal disturbances
Panhypopituitarism
Drugs and toxins
Environmental toxins (organophosphates, heavy metals, carbon monoxide)
Drug or alcohol intoxication and withdrawal
Adverse effects of prescription and over-the-counter medications

Source. Adapted from Rosse RB, Deutsch LH, Deutsch SI: "Medical Assessment and Laboratory Testing in Psychiatry," in *Kaplan and Sadock's Comprehensive Textbook of Psychiatry,* 7th Edition, Volume 1. Edited by Sadock BJ, Sadock VA. Baltimore, MD, Lippincott Williams & Wilkins, 1999, pp. 732–754; Wallach J: *Interpretation of Diagnostic Tests,* 5th Edition. Boston, MA, Little, Brown, 1992.

A complete psychiatric assessment, including a medical and psychiatric history, physical examination, and mental status examination, must be conducted before the initiation of any clinical and diagnostic testing. Such initial assessments will guide the clinician in his or her choices for relevant, cost-effective laboratory testing. Laboratory costs accounted for 10%–12% of total health care costs in 1990, and unnecessary tests should be avoided if they have little or no impact on the patient's treatment and outcome (Sheline and Kehr 1990). In this chapter we describe a systematic approach to the screening and diagnosis of the neuropsychiatric patient through the application of screening laboratory testing, and we highlight the usefulness of such testing in different clinical situations in neuropsychiatry. We also provide a brief overview of promising research on the use of genetic testing and biomarkers for the assessment of patients with neuropsychiatric disorders.

Screening Patients for Neuropsychiatric Disorders

Screening Laboratory Testing

At present there are no consensus guidelines for the initial laboratory screening of psychiatric patients without other known medical illnesses. Clinicians must be guided by the history, physical examination, and mental status examination and by their own clinical judgment to decide what tests are appropriate to obtain. Some studies of patient populations with general medical illnesses have shown that the history and review of systems obtained from the patient are superior to the physical examination in the diagnosis and management of patients and that laboratory testing is the least helpful (Barnes et al. 1983; Hampton et al. 1975). Other studies, however, indicate that there is little relationship between physical complaints and the presence of physical disease (Honig et al. 1991; Koran et al. 1989). Many studies have been conducted to investigate the utility of screening laboratory testing in the psychiatric patient, although most of these are retrospective studies that draw from varied patient populations

(Barnes et al. 1983; Catalano et al. 2001; Dolan and Mushlin 1985; Hall et al. 1980, 1981; Mookhoek and Sterrenburg-vdNieuwegiessen 1998; Sheline and Kehr 1990; White and Barraclough 1989; Willett and King 1977). In addition to a careful history and review of systems, as well as a thorough physical examination, psychiatric patients without other medical illnesses will benefit from a few screening tests such as serum glucose concentration, blood urea nitrogen concentration, creatinine clearance, and urinalysis (Anfinson and Kathol 1992). More extensive screening panels appear to be unnecessary. Screening of female psychiatric patients older than 50 years of age, especially those with mood symptoms, may be justified due to a high prevalence of hypothyroidism in the patients. Thyroid screening of men and younger women, among whom the prevalence of thyroid dysfunction is estimated to be 0.1%, should be limited to patients with two or more clinical signs of hypothyroidism (Anfinson and Stoudemire 2000).

No studies have been conducted to investigate this issue specifically for patients with neuropsychiatric illnesses. Several authors, however, have made a case for more extensive screening of several categories of patients: elderly individuals, institutionalized persons, persons of low socioeconomic status, individuals with a high degree of self-neglect, persons with alcohol or drug dependence, and those with cognitive impairment or fluctuating mental status (Anfinson and Kathol 1992; Hall et al. 1978; Koran et al. 1989; Sox et al. 1989). Given that individuals with neuropsychiatric illnesses often fall into these categories, a broader battery of tests will likely be appropriate for the workup of a patient who is being assessed for a neuropsychiatric disorder. Because screening laboratory tests will vary according to the patient's clinical presentation, the clinical situation (outpatient clinic vs. emergency room vs. inpatient setting) and concomitant medical illnesses, there is no such thing as routine screening laboratory tests for patients with putative neuropsychiatric conditions. Table 4–2 presents a list of screening laboratory tests that clinicians often use during the initial evaluation of a neuropsychiatric patient.

Table 4–2. Screening laboratory tests useful in the workup of neuropsychiatric patients

Type	Diagnostic test	Reference range	Clinical indication	Diagnostic considerations
Hematological studies	Coombs' test, direct and indirect	Positive/negative	Hemolytic anemias secondary to psychiatric medications	Evaluation of drug-induced hemolytic anemias, such as those secondary to administration of chlorpromazine, phenytoin, levodopa, and methyldopa
	Ferritin, serum	38–384 ng/mL	Cognitive/ neuropsychiatric workup	Decreased: iron-deficiency anemia; most sensitive test Elevated: anemias other than iron-deficiency
	Folate Plasma Red cell	 3.1–12.4 ng/mL 186–645 ng/mL	Alcohol abuse	Utilized in vitamin B_{12} deficiencies associated with psychosis, paranoia, fatigue, agitation, dementia, delirium
	Hemoglobin	Male: 14–18 g/dL Female: 12–16 g/dL	Cognitive/ neuropsychiatric workup	Decreased: alcohol abuse, cirrhosis, liver disease Elevated: polycythemias
	Hematocrit	Male: 41–51 g/dL Female: 37–47 g/dL	Cognitive/ neuropsychiatric workup	

Table 4–2. Screening laboratory tests useful in the workup of neuropsychiatric patients *(continued)*

Type	Diagnostic test	Reference range	Clinical indication	Diagnostic considerations
Hematological studies *(continued)*	Iron, serum	60–160 μg/dL	Cognitive/neuropsychiatric workup	Decreased: iron-deficiency anemia, other normochromic anemias
	Iron-binding capacity	220–420 μg/dL	Cognitive/neuropsychiatric workup	Decreased: hemochromatosis, liver cirrhosis, thalassemia Elevated: iron-deficiency anemia, acute and chronic blood loss, acute liver damage
	Mean corpuscular volume	87 ± 5 μm^3	Alcohol abuse	Elevated: alcoholism and vitamin B_{12} and folate deficiency
	Partial thromboplastin time (PTT)	21–32 seconds	Treatment with antipsychotics, heparin	Monitor anticoagulant therapy Elevated: in presence of lupus anticoagulant and anticardiolipin antibodies
	Platelet count	150–400 K/μL	Use of psychotropic medications	Decreased by certain psychotropic medications (carbamazepine, clozapine, phenothiazines)

Table 4–2. Screening laboratory tests useful in the workup of neuropsychiatric patients *(continued)*

Type	Diagnostic test	Reference range	Clinical indication	Diagnostic considerations
Hematological studies *(continued)*	Porphobilinogen (PBG) deaminase (erythrocyte uroporphyrinogen-1-synthetase)	2.1–4.3 mU/g Hgb	Porphyrias	Decreased: porphyria-synthesizing enzyme in red blood cells (RBCs) in patients with acute intermittent porphyria
	Prothrombin time	8.2–10.3 seconds	Cognitive/medical workup	Elevated: significant liver damage (cirrhosis)
	Reticulocyte count	0.5%–1.5%	Cognitive/medical workup	Decreased: megaloblastic or iron deficiency anemia and anemia of chronic disease, alcoholism Indicator of effective RBC production
	White blood cell count	3.8–9.8 × $10^3/\mu L$	Use of psychiatric medications	Leukopenia and agranulocytosis associated with certain psychotropic medications (phenothiazines, carbamazepine, clozapine) Leukocytosis associated with lithium and neuroleptic malignant syndrome

Table 4–2. Screening laboratory tests useful in the workup of neuropsychiatric patients *(continued)*

Type	Diagnostic test	Reference range	Clinical indication	Diagnostic considerations
Serum chemistries/ vitamins	Acid phosphatase	0–0.7 IU/L	Cognitive/medical workup	Elevated: prostate cancer, benign prostatic hypertrophy, excessive platelet destruction, bone disease
	Alanine aminotransferase/ serum glutamic-pyruvic transaminase	7–53 IU/L	Neuropsychiatric workup	Elevated: hepatitis, cirrhosis, liver metastasis Decreased: vitamin B_6/ pyridoxine deficiency
	Albumin	3.6–5.0 g/dL	Cognitive/medical workup	Elevated: dehydration
	Aldolase	1.5–8.1 U/L	Eating disorders, schizophrenia	Elevated: patients who abuse ipecac (e.g., bulimic patients), some patients with schizophrenia
	Alkaline phosphatase	38–126 IU/L	Cognitive/ neuropsychiatric workup Use of psychiatric medications	Elevated: Paget's disease, hyperparathyroidism, hepatic disease, liver metastases, heart failure, phenothiazine use Decreased: pernicious anemia (vitamin B_{12} deficiency)

Table 4–2. Screening laboratory tests useful in the workup of neuropsychiatric patients *(continued)*

Type	Diagnostic test	Reference range	Clinical indication	Diagnostic considerations
Serum chemistries/ vitamins ***(continued)***	Ammonia	9–3 mmol/L	Cognitive/ neuropsychiatric workup	Elevated: hepatic encephalopathy, liver failure, Reye's syndrome; increases with gastrointestinal hemorrhage and severe congestive heart failure
	Amylase	25–115 IU/L	Eating disorders	May be elevated in bulimia nervosa
	Aspartate aminotransferase	11–47 IU/L	Cognitive/ neuropsychiatric workup	Elevated: heart failure, hepatic disease, pancreatitis, eclampsia, cerebral damage, alcoholism Decreased: pyridoxine (vitamin B_6) deficiency and terminal stages of liver disease
	Bicarbonate	21–29 mEq/L	Panic disorder Eating disorders	Decreased: hyperventilation syndrome, panic disorder, anabolic steroid abuse May be elevated in patients with bulimia nervosa or in laxative abuse or psychogenic vomiting

Table 4–2. Screening laboratory tests useful in the workup of neuropsychiatric patients *(continued)*

Type	Diagnostic test	Reference range	Clinical indication	Diagnostic considerations
Serum chemistries/ vitamins ***(continued)***	Bilirubin	0.3–1.1 mg/dL	Cognitive/ neuropsychiatric workup	Elevated: hepatic disease
	Blood urea nitrogen (BUN)	17–45 mg/dL	Delirium	Elevated: renal disease, dehydration
	Calcium	8.6–10.3 mg/dL	Cognitive/ neuropsychiatric workup Mood disorders Psychosis Eating disorders	Elevated: hyperparathyroidism, bone metastases Elevation associated with delirium, depression, psychosis Decreased: hypoparathyroidism, renal failure Decrease associated with depression, irritability, delirium, chronic laxative abuse
	Chloride	97–110 mmol/L	Eating disorders Panic disorder	Decreased: patients with bulimia, psychogenic vomiting
	CO_2 content (plasma)	22–32 mmol/L	Cognitive/ neuropsychiatric workup Delirium	Mild elevation in hyperventilation syndrome, panic disorder

Table 4–2. Screening laboratory tests useful in the workup of neuropsychiatric patients *(continued)*

Type	Diagnostic test	Reference range	Clinical indication	Diagnostic considerations
Serum chemistries/ vitamins *(continued)*	Creatine phosphokinase	≤150 U/L	Delirium	Elevated: neuroleptic malignant syndrome, intramuscular injection rhabdomyolysis (secondary to substance abuse), patients in restraint, patients experiencing dystonic reactions; asymptomatic elevations with use of antipsychotic drugs
	Creatinine (Cr)	0.8–1.8 g/day	Cognitive/ neuropsychiatric workup	Elevated: renal disease (see BUN)
	Gamma-glutamyl transpeptidase (GGT), serum	11–50 IU/L 7–32 IU/L	Alcohol abuse	Elevated: alcohol abuse, cirrhosis, liver disease
	Glucose	65–109 mg/dL	Panic attacks Anxiety Delirium Depression	Very high fasting blood sugar associated with delirium Very low fasting blood sugar associated with delirium, agitation, panic attacks, anxiety, depression

Table 4–2. Screening laboratory tests useful in the workup of neuropsychiatric patients *(continued)*

Type	Diagnostic test	Reference range	Clinical indication	Diagnostic considerations
Serum chemistries/ vitamins ***(continued)***	Lactate dehydrogenase	100–250 IU/L	Cognitive/ neuropsychiatric workup	Elevated: myocardial infarction, pulmonary infarction, hepatic disease, renal infarction, seizures, cerebral damage, megaloblastic (pernicious) anemia. Factitious elevations secondary to rough handling of blood specimen tube
	Magnesium, serum	1.7–2.4 mg/dL	Alcohol abuse Cognitive/ neuropsychiatric workup	Decreased: alcoholism; low levels associated with agitation, delirium, seizures
	Phosphorus, serum	2.5–4.5 mg/dL	Cognitive/ neuropsychiatric workup	Increased: acute porphyria

Table 4–2. Screening laboratory tests useful in the workup of neuropsychiatric patients *(continued)*

Type	Diagnostic test	Reference range	Clinical indication	Diagnostic considerations
Serum chemistries/ vitamins *(continued)*	Potassium	3.3–4.9 mmol/L	Cognitive/ neuropsychiatric workup	Increased: hyperkalemic acidosis; increase is associated with anxiety in cardiac arrhythmia
			Eating disorders	Decreased: cirrhosis, metabolic alkalosis, laxative abuse, diuretic abuse; decrease is common in bulimic patients and in psychogenic vomiting, anabolic steroid abuse
	Protein, total	6.5–8.5 g/dL	Cognitive/ neuropsychiatric workup	Increased: multiple myeloma, myxedema, lupus
	Sodium	135–145 mmol/L	Cognitive/ neuropsychiatric workup	Decreased: water intoxication; syndrome of inappropriate antidiuretic hormone secretion
				Decreased: hypoadrenalism, myxedema, congestive heart failure, diarrhea, polydipsia, use of carbamazepine, anabolic steroids

Table 4–2. Screening laboratory tests useful in the workup of neuropsychiatric patients *(continued)*

Type	Diagnostic test	Reference range	Clinical indication	Diagnostic considerations
Serum chemistries/ vitamins *(continued)*	Vitamin A, serum	360–1,200 mg/L	Depression Delirium	Hypervitaminosis A is associated with a variety of mental status changes, headache
	Vitamin B_{12}, serum	200–1,100 pg/mL	Cognitive/ neuropsychiatric workup Dementia Mood disorder	Part of workup of megaloblastic anemia and dementia B_{12} deficiency is associated with psychosis, paranoia, fatigue, agitation, dementia, delirium Often associated with chronic alcohol abuse
	Zinc, serum	65–2561 μg/dL	Cognitive/ neuropsychiatric workup	Evaluate possible deficiency or toxicity
Endocrine studies	Adrenocorticotrophic hormone	<60 pg/mL	Cognitive/ neuropsychiatric workup	Changes with steroid abuse; may be elevated in seizures, psychosis, and Cushing's disease and in response to stress
	Human chorionic gonadotropin beta (β-hCG)	Negative	Pregnancy test	Prior to initiation of teratogenic psychotropic medications

Table 4–2. Screening laboratory tests useful in the workup of neuropsychiatric patients *(continued)*

Type	Diagnostic test	Reference range	Clinical indication	Diagnostic considerations
Endocrine studies ***(continued)***	Cortisol	6–30 mg/dL	Cognitive/ neuropsychiatric workup Mood disorders	Excess levels may indicate Cushing's disease; associated with anxiety, depression, and a variety of other conditions
	Catecholamines, urinary and plasma	<540 μg/day	Panic attacks Anxiety	Elevated: pheochromocytoma
	Estrogens, total	Male: 29–127 pg/mL Female: 35–650 pg/mL (varies over the menstrual cycle)	Mood disorder	Decreased: menopausal depression and premenstrual syndrome; variable changes in anxiety
	Follicle-stimulating hormone	Male: 1.1–13.5 mIU/mL Female: 0.4–22.6 mIU/mL (varies over the menstrual cycle)	Depression	High normal in anorexia nervosa, higher values in postmenopausal women; low levels in patients with panhypopituitarism

Table 4–2. Screening laboratory tests useful in the workup of neuropsychiatric patients *(continued)*

Type	Diagnostic test	Reference range	Clinical indication	Diagnostic considerations
Endocrine studies *(continued)*	Growth hormone (GH)	Adult male: <1 ng/mL Adult female: <10 ng/mL	Depression Anxiety Schizophrenia	Blunted GH response to insulin-induced hypoglycemia in depressed patients; increased GH response to dopamine agonist challenge in schizophrenic patients Elevated in some anorexia patients
	Luteinizing hormone	Male: 1.4–7.7 mIU/mL Female: 1.6–62.0 mIU/mL (varies over the menstrual cycle)	Depression	Decreased: patients with panhypopituitarism Decrease associated with depression
	Parathyroid hormone	12–72 pg/mL	Anxiety Cognitive/neuropsychiatric workup	Low level causes hypocalcemia and anxiety Dysregulation associated with wide variety of organic mental disorders

Table 4–2. Screening laboratory tests useful in the workup of neuropsychiatric patients *(continued)*

Type	Diagnostic test	Reference range	Clinical indication	Diagnostic considerations
Endocrine studies *(continued)*	Prolactin	Male: 1.6–18.8 ng/mL Female: 1.4–24.2 ng/mL	Use of antipsychotic medications Cocaine use Pseudoseizures	Antipsychotics, by decreasing dopamine, increase prolactin synthesis and release, especially in women Elevated: cocaine withdrawal Lack of prolactin elevation after seizure suggestive of pseudoseizure
	Testosterone, serum	Male: 270–1,070 ng/dL Female: 6–86 ng/dL	Impotence, inhibited sexual desire	Elevated: anabolic steroid abuse May be decreased in impotence and inhibited sexual desire Used in follow-up of sex offenders treated with medroxyprogesterone Decreased: medroxyprogesterone treatment

Table 4–2. Screening laboratory tests useful in the workup of neuropsychiatric patients *(continued)*

Type	Diagnostic test	Reference range	Clinical indication	Diagnostic considerations
Endocrine studies *(continued)*	Thyroid function tests		Cognitive/ neuropsychiatric workup	Detection of hypothyroidism or hyperthyroidism
	Thyroid-stimulating hormone (TSH)	2–11 μU/mL	Depression	Abnormalities can be associated with depression, anxiety, psychosis, dementia, delirium, or lithium treatment
	Thyroxine (T_4)	4–11 μg/dL		
	Triiodothyronine (T_3)	75–220 ng/dL		
	Thyroxine-binding globulin capacity	12–28 μg/dL		
	T_3 resin uptake	25%–35%		
Autoimmune studies	Antinuclear antibody	Negative at 1:10 dilution	Cognitive/ neuropsychiatric workup	Most sensitive test for systemic lupus erythematosus (SLE) (detects up to 95% of cases; specificity is low in rheumatic diseases in general [50%]) Elevated: erythematosus (SLE) and drug-induced lupus (e.g., secondary to phenothiazines, anticonvulsants); SLE can be associated with delirium, psychosis, mood disorders

Table 4–2. Screening laboratory tests useful in the workup of neuropsychiatric patients *(continued)*

Type	Diagnostic test	Reference range	Clinical indication	Diagnostic considerations
Autoimmune studies ***(continued)***	Anti–double-stranded DNA antibody	Negative at 1:10 dilution	Cognitive/neuropsychiatric workup	Positive in 40%–80% of SLE patients High titers characteristic of SLE; low titers in other rheumatic diseases
	Erythrocyte sedimentation rate	<50 mm/hour	Cognitive/neuropsychiatric workup	Elevated: nonspecific indicator of infectious, inflammatory, autoimmune, or malignant disease Sometimes recommended in the evaluation of anorexia nervosa
	Lupus anticoagulant	Negative	Use of phenothiazines	An antiphospholipid antibody, which has been described in some patients using phenothiazines, especially chlorpromazine; often associated with elevated PTT; associated with anticardiolipin antibodies
	Rheumatoid factor	0.0–20.0 IU/mL	Neuropsychiatric workup	Use in evaluation of stroke in young person or vasculitis

Table 4–2. Screening laboratory tests useful in the workup of neuropsychiatric patients *(continued)*

Type	Diagnostic test	Reference range	Clinical indication	Diagnostic considerations
Cerebrospinal fluid (CSF) studies	Acid-fast bacilli stain	None detected	Neuropsychiatric workup	Useful for diagnosis of tuberculous meningitis
	Cell count, CSF	0–2 white blood cells (WBCs)	Neuropsychiatric workup	Lymphocytes present in tuberculous meningitis
		0–5 RBCs		Polymorphonuclear neutrophils present in bacterial meningitis
	Culture and sensitivities		Neuropsychiatric workup	For evaluation of bacterial meningitis/encephalitis
	Glucose, CSF	65–109 mg/dL	Neuropsychiatric workup	Decreased: bacterial, tuberculous and fungal meningitis
	Immunoglobulin G (IgG)	700–1,450 mg/dL	Neuropsychiatric workup	Elevated in 70% of multiple sclerosis (MS) patients
	Myelin basic protein	0.07–4.10 ng/mL	Neuropsychiatric workup	Elevated in 70%–90% of MS patients during an acute exacerbation; also elevated in other demyelinating diseases

Table 4–2. Screening laboratory tests useful in the workup of neuropsychiatric patients *(continued)*

Type	Diagnostic test	Reference range	Clinical indication	Diagnostic considerations
Cerebrospinal fluid (CSF) studies *(continued)*	Protein electrophoresis (CSF and serum) Prealbumin Albumin Oligoclonal bands Alpha-1, alpha-2, beta, gamma		Neuropsychiatric workup	Oligoclonal bands positive in 85%–95% of patients with definite MS; most sensitive marker of MS Use in evaluation of inflammatory and hypercoagulable states
	Opening pressure	<7 mm Hg (100 mm water)	Neuropsychiatric workup	Elevated: in pseudotumor cerebri, meningitis, subarachnoid hemorrhage, or other head trauma
	Protein, CSF	6.5–8.5 g/dL	Neuropsychiatric workup	Elevated: bacterial, tuberculous, and fungal meningitis Must obtain serum protein levels as reference
Serological studies	Cytomegalovirus (CMV) antibodies, serum	Negative CMV IgG: <4.0 AU/mL CMV IgM: <0.7 TV	Altered mental status/ neuropsychiatric workup	CMV can produce anxiety, confusion, mood disorders CMV IgG and immunoglobulin M (IgM)

Table 4–2. Screening laboratory tests useful in the workup of neuropsychiatric patients *(continued)*

Type	Diagnostic test	Reference range	Clinical indication	Diagnostic considerations
Serological studies *(continued)*	Epstein-Barr virus (EBV), serum and CSF	Positive/negative	Cognitive/neuropsychiatric workup Anxiety Mood disorders	Part of herpesvirus group EBV is the causative agent for infectious mononucleosis, which can present with depression, fatigue, and personality change EBV may be associated with a chronic mononucleosis-like syndrome consisting of chronic depression and fatigue
	Hepatitis antibody	Positive/negative	Mood disorders Cognitive/neuropsychiatric workup	Less severe, better prognosis than hepatitis B; may present with anorexia, depression
	Hepatitis B surface antigen, hepatitis B core antigen	Positive/negative	Mood disorders Cognitive/neuropsychiatric workup	Active hepatitis B infection indicates greater degree of infectivity and of progression to chronic liver disease

Table 4–2. Screening laboratory tests useful in the workup of neuropsychiatric patients *(continued)*

Type	Diagnostic test	Reference range	Clinical indication	Diagnostic considerations
Serological studies *(continued)*	Hepatitis C core antibody	Positive/negative	Mood disorders	High rates of depression related to interferon treatment
			Cognitive/neuropsychiatric workup	
	Human immunodeficiency virus–1 p24 antigen, serum	Positive/negative	Altered mental status/neuropsychiatric workup	Positive enzyme-linked immunosorbent assay confirmed via Western blot or immunofluorescence assay
	Lyme titer, serum	Negative	Altered mental status	Evaluation of meningitis due to Lyme disease *(Borrelia burgdorferi)*
				Elevated: IgM and IgG antibodies
				Suspected cause of meningitis with elevated lymphocytes, elevated protein, and IgG oligoclonal bands in CSF
	Syphilis test (rapid plasma reagin test, venereal disease research laboratory slide test), serum, CSF	Nonreactive	Neuropsychiatric workup	Positive in syphilis

Table 4–2. Screening laboratory tests useful in the workup of neuropsychiatric patients *(continued)*

Type	Diagnostic test	Reference range	Clinical indication	Diagnostic considerations
Urine tests	Myoglobin	0–1 mg/L	Phenothiazine use Substance abuse Use of restraints	Elevated: neuroleptic malignant syndrome; phencyclidine, cocaine, or lysergic acid diethylamide intoxication; and in patients in restraints
	Urinalysis		Cognitive/neuropsychiatric workup Pretreatment workup of lithium Drug screening	Provides clues to cause of various cognitive disorders (assessing general appearance, pH, specific gravity, bilirubin, glucose, blood, ketones, protein, etc.); specific gravity may be affected by lithium
	Specific gravity	1.005–1.030		
	pH	5.0–8.5		
	Protein	Negative		
	Glucose	Negative		
	Occult blood	Negative		
	Ketones	Negative		
	Bilirubin	Negative		
	Nitrite	Negative		
	Urobilinogen	0.1–1.0		
	Microscopic	Females: ≤4 WBCs/hpf, ≤2 RBCs/hpf Males: ≤1 WBC/hpf, ≤1 RBC/hpf		

Table 4–2. Screening laboratory tests useful in the workup of neuropsychiatric patients *(continued)*

Type	Diagnostic test	Reference range	Clinical indication	Diagnostic considerations
Urine tests *(continued)*	Urine porphyrins		Altered mental status	Elevated: acute intermittent porphyria, especially during acute attack
	Uroporphyrin	0–4 μmol/mol Cr		
	Coproporphyrin	0–22 μmol/mol Cr		
	Porphobilinogen	0–8.8 μmol/L		
	Urine catecholamines		Altered mental status, anxiety	Elevated: pheochromocytoma
	Epinephrine	2–24 μg/d		
	Norepinephrine	15–100 μg/d		
	Total (epi+norepi)	26–161 μg/d		
	Dopamine	52–480 μg/d		
	Urine VMA	0–7.0 μg/d		
	Urine metanephrines			Metanephrines most reliable screening test for pheochromocytoma
	Metanephrine	35–460 μg/d		
	Normetanephrine	110–1050 μg/d		
Toxicology	Alcohol		Altered mental status, anxiety	Elevated blood alcohol level varies by state law >0.08%–0.15% Tolerance is likely if blood alcohol level is >0.10% but intoxication symptoms are absent Elevated GGT and liver function tests (LFTs)

Table 4–2. Screening laboratory tests useful in the workup of neuropsychiatric patients *(continued)*

Type	Diagnostic test	Reference range	Clinical indication	Diagnostic considerations
Toxicology *(continued)*	Amphetamines	Positive/negative	Altered mental status	
	Barbiturates	Positive/negative	Altered mental status	
	Benzodiazepines	Positive/negative	Altered mental status Suicide attempts	
	Caffeine	Positive/negative	Anxiety/panic disorder	Evaluation of patients with suspected caffeinism
	Cannabis	Positive/negative	Altered mental status	
	Cocaine	Positive/negative	Altered mental status	Elevated levels of benzoylecgonine (metabolite) present
	Hallucinogens	Positive/negative	Altered mental status	
	Inhalants	Positive/negative	Altered mental status	
	Nicotine	Positive/negative	Anxiety Nicotine addiction	Evaluation of anxiety in smokers Elevated levels of cotinine (metabolite) can be detected in blood, saliva, or urine
	Opiates/narcotics	Positive/negative	Altered mental status	
	Phencyclidine	Positive/negative	Altered mental status	Elevated glutamic-oxaloacetic transaminase and creatine phosphokinase

Table 4–2. Screening laboratory tests useful in the workup of neuropsychiatric patients *(continued)*

Type	Diagnostic test	Reference range	Clinical indication	Diagnostic considerations
Toxicology *(continued)*	Salicylates		Organic hallucinosis Suicide attempts	Toxic levels may be seen in suicide attempts High levels may cause organic hallucinosis
Other diagnostic tests and procedures	CO_2 inhalation, sodium bicarbonate infusion		Anxiety/panic disorder	Provocative test Panic attacks induced in subgroup of patients
	Doppler ultrasound		Impotence Cognitive/neuropsychiatric workup	Carotid occlusion, transient ischemic attack, reduced penile blood flow in impotence
	Echocardiogram		Panic disorder	10%–40% of patients with panic disorder have mitral valve prolapse

Table 4–2. Screening laboratory tests useful in the workup of neuropsychiatric patients *(continued)*

Type	Diagnostic test	Reference range	Clinical indication	Diagnostic considerations
Other diagnostic tests and procedures *(continued)*	Electroencephalogram		Cognitive/ neuropsychiatric workup	Evaluation of seizures, brain death, lesions;
				Shortened rapid eye movement (REM) latency in depression
				High-voltage activity in excitement, functional nonorganic cases (e.g., dissociative states), alpha activity present in the background, which responds to auditory and visual stimuli
				Biphasic or triphasic slow bursts seen in dementia of Creutzfeldt-Jacob disease
	Holter monitor		Panic disorder	Evaluation of patients with panic disorder who have palpitations and other cardiac symptoms

Table 4–2. Screening laboratory tests useful in the workup of neuropsychiatric patients *(continued)*

Type	Diagnostic test	Reference range	Clinical indication	Diagnostic considerations
Other diagnostic tests and procedures *(continued)*	Nocturnal penile tumescence		Impotence	Quantification of penile circumference changes, penile rigidity, frequency of penile tumescence Evaluation of erectile function during sleep Erections associated with REM sleep Helpful in differentiation between organic and functional causes of impotence

Note. Reference values are provided in conventional units; values shown are for adults and may vary between laboratories. VMA = vanillylmandelic acid.

Source. Adapted from Alpay M, Park L: "Laboratory Tests and Diagnostic Procedures," in *Psychiatry: Update and Board Preparation.* Edited by Stern TA, Herman JB. New York, McGraw-Hill, 2000, pp. 251–265; Anfinson TJ, Stoudemire A: "Laboratory and Neuroendocrine Assessment in Medical-Psychiatric Patients," in *Psychiatric Care of the Medical Patient,* 2nd Edition. Edited by Stoudemire A, Fogel BS, Greenberg DB. New York, Oxford University Press, 2000, pp. 119–145; Fadem B, Simring S: *High Yield Psychiatry.* Baltimore, MD, Williams & Wilkins, 1998; Methodist Health Care System: *Laboratory Medicine Handbook,* 4th Edition. Hudson, OH, Lexi-Comp, 2001; Rosse RB, Deutsch LH, Deutsch SI: "Medical Assessment and Laboratory Testing in Psychiatry," in *Kaplan and Sadock's Comprehensive Textbook of Psychiatry,* 7th Edition, Volume 1. Edited by Sadock BJ, Sadock VA. Baltimore, MD, Lippincott Williams & Wilkins, 1999, pp. 732–754; and Wallach J: *Interpretation of Diagnostic Tests,* 5th Edition. Boston, MA, Little, Brown, 1992. Used with permission.

Screening Chest Radiographs

Several studies have involved retrospective review of the utility of the screening chest radiograph in the evaluation of psychiatric patients. Data from several studies show that there is little evidence that a routine chest radiograph will yield beneficial information for a patient without respiratory or neurological symptoms (Brown 1995; Gomez-Gil et al. 2002; Harms and Hermans 1994; Hughes and Barraclough 1980; Liston et al. 1979; Mookhoek and Sterrenburg-vdNieuwegiessen 1998). These data, in addition to the knowledge that there are currently no screening guidelines for chest radiographs in the general population, indicate that the *routine* screening chest radiograph is not indicated for a person who is being evaluated for the presence of a psychiatric disorder. However, chest radiographs are clearly indicated for specific clinical situations in the assessment of a patient with a neuropsychiatric disorder. For example, if an elderly patient had the sudden onset of fever, shortness of breath, chest pain, and delirium, a chest radiograph should be ordered on an emergency basis.

Screening Electrocardiograms

Several studies have shown that the routine performance of screening electrocardiograms (ECGs) on young, medically healthy psychiatric patients who do not have cardiovascular symptoms is unnecessary (Hollister 1995). However, studies differ regarding the importance of electrocardiography in the elderly, with many finding an increased prevalence of electrocardiographic abnormalities in people over age 50. Furthermore, these studies differ with regard to the clinical importance or outcome that these abnormalities might have for the patient's health (Hall et al. 1980; Harms and Hermans 1994; Hollister 1995; Mookhoek and Sterrenburg-vdNieuwegiessen 1998). All agree that regardless of age, an ECG is indicated when the history, review of systems, or findings from the physical examination suggest cardiovascular disease or if a patient is initiating treatment with a psychotropic drug, such as a tricyclic antidepressant (TCA) or an antipsychotic, that is known to alter cardiac function or increase cardiac conduction times.

Overall Role of Screening

The consensus of studies evaluating the role and value of laboratory testing is that patients who have psychiatric signs and symptoms but who do not exhibit other physical complaints or symptoms will benefit from a small screening battery that includes serum glucose concentration, blood urea nitrogen concentration, creatinine clearance, and urinalysis. Female patients over age 50 will also benefit from a screening thyroid-stimulating hormone (TSH) test regardless of the presence or absence of mood symptoms. Broader screening panels are generally unnecessary and costly. However, because the neuropsychiatric patient, by definition, often has neurological and medical conditions that affect mood, cognition, memory, and behavior, a much broader use of laboratory testing is often warranted. Because there are no existing studies of the utility of laboratory testing specific to neuropsychiatric patients, laboratory testing should be obtained for the following purposes: 1) the initial assessment of possible medical and neurological etiologies of signs and symptoms that indicate the presence of neuropsychiatric disorder (e.g., disorientation, confusion, memory impairment, visual hallucinations); 2) follow-up evaluation of medication side effects, drug levels, and response; and 3) the assessment of neuropsychiatric symptoms that might be the result of alcohol, prescribed medications, substances of abuse, poisons, and toxins.

Specific Clinical Indications for Laboratory Testing in Neuropsychiatry

The clinical conditions described below indicate that a more extensive laboratory workup is necessary.

New-Onset Psychosis

A careful neuropsychiatric evaluation is important for a patient with a first episode of psychosis, because there are many medical and neurological causes of psychosis. Routine screening tests often include serum chemistries including sodium, potassium, chloride, carbon dioxide, blood urea nitrogen, and creatinine; liver function tests such as total protein, total and direct bilirubin, serum aspartate transaminase/glutamic-oxaloacetic transaminase, and alanine aminotransferase/serum glutamic-pyruvic transaminase; complete blood count (CBC) with platelets and differential; TSH, syphilis, and human immunodeficiency virus (HIV) serology; serum alcohol level; urinalysis; and urine toxicology screen for drugs of abuse. Other tests to consider during the initial workup include neuroimaging and electroencephalography, which are covered in other chapters of this volume. If appropriate, the clinician should also consider ordering a urine pregnancy test and baseline ECG, especially if he or she is planning initiation of or change in antipsychotic medication.

If these initial tests do not immediately yield an etiology, the clinician may also consider a lumbar puncture to analyze cerebrospinal fluid (CSF) for the presence of red and white blood cells, protein, and glucose; opening pressure; and bacterial culture and viral serologies. Antinuclear antibodies, rheumatoid factor, erythrocyte sedimentation rate, urine porphyrins, blood cultures, and assays for heavy metals (manganese and mercury) and bromides are other tests to consider. There are many causes of psychosis that must be ruled out, including central nervous system (CNS) or systemic infections, temporal lobe epilepsy, substance intoxication and withdrawal, metabolic or endocrine disorders, CNS tumors, and heavy metal poisoning.

Mood Disturbance: Depressive or Manic Symptoms

A thorough laboratory screening is also recommended for the evaluation of adult patients with new-onset mood symptoms such as depression or mania. Tests might include TSH concentration, serum chemistries, CBC, urinalysis, and urine toxicology screen for drugs of abuse. If appropriate, the clinician should also consider ordering a urine pregnancy test and ECG, especially if he or she is considering starting a mood-stabilizing medication. Measuring levels of therapeutic drugs can be helpful to confirm the presence of a drug if nonadherence is suspected or if therapeutic effect is not obtained, to determine whether toxicity may be contributing to the patient's clinical presentation, or to determine whether drug interactions have altered the desired therapeutic levels (Wallach 1992). Serum trough levels of mood stabilizers (such as lithium, valproate, or carbamazepine) and TCAs can be obtained to monitor therapeutic response in accordance with therapeutic levels. Similarly, drug levels of TCAs may also be obtained, although it is unclear whether blood levels of antidepressants correlate with therapeutic response (Hyman et al. 1995). However, TCA drug levels can be useful to confirm the presence of the drug or to confirm extremely high serum levels. Please see "Monitoring Medications" later for further information regarding therapeutic drug levels. Neuroimaging and electroencephalography are often helpful as well in understanding the etiology of a patient's mood symptoms. Multiple neurological and medical disorders have mood manifestations, which may often be the presenting complaint. For example, stroke, seizure disorders, Parkinson's disease, and thyroid and other endocrine abnormalities may all present with depression, mania or hypomania, or psychosis as the primary complaint, with only subtle physical and cognitive manifestations that may be missed by cursory clinical examination. Further workup with structural and sometimes functional imaging and electroencephalography can often prevent disastrous outcomes by uncovering the medical or neurological etiology, thus providing the patient with effective treatment or prophylaxis against further episodes.

Anxiety

The initial workup for anxiety symptoms should include serum chemistries, serum glucose, and TSH and other endocrine measures. Many different medical and neurological diseases can manifest with anxiety, including angina and myocardial infarction; mitral valve prolapse; substance intoxication and withdrawal; and metabolic and endocrine disorders such as thyroid abnormalities, pheochromocytoma, and hypoglycemia. Cardiac workup is important, because cardiac symptoms may masquerade as panic attacks (or vice versa) and are often misdiagnosed as such, especially in female patients. Therefore, electrocardiography, Holter monitoring, stress test, and echocardiography are just a few cardiac examinations that may be necessary. Respiratory function should also be evaluated with a chest radiograph or pulmonary function tests to rule out chronic obstructive pulmonary disease as a contributory factor. Other tests to consider if one has clinical suspicion include electroencephalography, urine porphyrins, and urine vanillylmandelic acid.

Altered Mental Status

Patients with a fluctuating mental status of acute onset most likely will have one or more underlying medical or neurological causes for their impaired consciousness. This often constitutes a medical emergency, and comprehensive laboratory and diagnostic testing is indicated on an emergency basis. In addition to a complete physical examination and as much history as can be obtained from the patient and ancillary sources, the clinician should order serum chemistries, CBC, erythrocyte sedimentation rate, HIV serology, urinalysis and urine toxicology, ECG, and chest radiograph. A computed tomographic scan, blood cultures, lumbar puncture with CSF analysis, and EEG can be helpful as well if they are clinically indicated. Many medical and neurological disorders can cause impairment in mental status. These include seizures, CNS and systemic infection, kidney or liver failure, cardiac arrhythmias, stroke, myocardial infarction, and substance intoxication and withdrawal.

Cognitive Decline and Dementia

Laboratory testing is a major component of the comprehensive evaluation of cognitive decline. The current American Academy of Neurology practice recommendations for evaluation of reversible causes of dementia include testing for vitamin B_{12} deficiency and hypothyroidism. Immunoassay for CSF 14-3-3 protein is useful for confirmation of clinical suspicions of Creutzfeldt-Jacob disease in a patient with rapidly progressive dementia and pathognomonic neurological symptoms (i.e., myoclonic jerks), although false-positive results can occur with other acute neurological conditions such as viral encephalitis, stroke, and paraneoplastic neurological disorders. These laboratory tests are recommended in addition to structural imaging (noncontrast head computed tomographic or magnetic resonance imaging studies) and evaluation of depression to rule out so-called pseudodementia, or dementia-like symptoms that stem from depression. Syphilis serology screening is not necessary in patients with dementia unless neurosyphilis is clinically suspected. Other imaging modalities—such as linear and volumetric imaging, single-photon emission computed tomography, and positron emission tomography—are not recommended at this time because there are insufficient data on the validity of these tests to diagnose illnesses that lead to cognitive disorders and dementia. There are no CSF or other biomarkers currently recommended for routine use in the diagnosis of dementia, although the utility of several tests is being investigated.

Mild Cognitive Impairment

There are no current clinical recommendations for the laboratory assessment of patients who have mild cognitive impairment but do not yet meet criteria for dementia. Patients with mild cognitive impairment are at high risk for developing dementia or Alzheimer's disease. However, the utility of diagnostic workup aside from cognitive screening is as yet unknown. Patients who have symptoms of mild cognitive impairment will likely benefit from a thyroid screen. Other laboratory tests typically ordered for the evaluation of dementia may be of use should signs and symptoms be elicited from the history, review of systems, or physical examination. For example, it may be useful to measure folate and vitamin B_{12} levels in a patient with mild cognitive impairment who has a long history of alcohol abuse or who is discovered to have peripheral neuropathy on the neurological examination.

Substance Abuse

In a study of 345 consecutive patients who presented to the emergency room of an urban teaching hospital with primary psychiatric complaints, 141 of these patients (41%) had positive urine toxicology screens for substances of abuse, and 90 (26%) had positive ethanol screens (Olshaker et al. 1997). Clearly, laboratory testing is essential to the evaluation, monitoring, and subsequent treatment of patients who abuse alcohol, prescribed addictive medications, or illicit drugs. Laboratory detection of drugs of abuse, as well as test results indicative of end-organ damage related to the abuse, can provide valuable hard evidence for the treating clinician to be informed and monitor his or her patient's progress. These data are also frequently useful in confronting the denial of substance abuse by the patient or his or her family. Laboratory testing can be conducted with blood and urine specimens or with saliva and hair samples. Urine specimens are typically preferred, because the detectable length of time that a particular drug of abuse and its metabolites are present is longer in urine than in blood. However, some substances, such as alcohol or barbiturates, are best detected in blood specimens. The length of time that a drug of abuse is detectable in the urine varies based on the amount and duration of substance consumed, kidney and liver function, and the specific drug itself. Laboratory methodologies vary. Usually an initial screening of blood and urine can provide a nonspecific but sensitive test for alcohol and other substances of abuse. If the screening tests yield a positive result, follow-up with more specific tests, including quantitative analyses, can be ordered for confirmation. Table 4–3 reviews common drugs of abuse, length of detection time, and common psychiatric manifestations of each.

Monitoring Medications

Measuring levels of therapeutic drugs to evaluate for toxicity and effective levels can be extremely helpful in the workup and treatment of the neuropsychiatric patient. Therapeutic drug monitoring should be used to confirm the presence and level of the drug if noncompliance is suspected, if the desired therapeutic effect is not obtained, or if signs or symptoms of toxicity occur; to determine whether toxicity may be contributing to the patient's clinical presentation; or to determine whether drug

Table 4–3. Substances of abuse

Agent	Toxic level	Urine detection time
Alcohol	300 mg/dL at any time or >100 g ingested	7–12 hours
Amphetamines		48 hours
Barbiturates	>6 μg/mL	24 hours (short-acting) 3 weeks (long-acting)
Benzodiazepines	Varies with medication Lorazepam: >25–100 mg Diazepam: >250 mg	3 days
Cannabis	50–200 μg/kg	4–6 weeks
Cocaine	>1.2 g	6–8 hours 2–4 days (metabolites)
Opiates	Varies with medication Heroin: >100–250 mg Codeine: >500–1,000 mg Morphine: > 50–100 μg/kg	2–3 days
Phencyclidine	>10–20 mg	1–2 weeks

Source. Adapted from Wallach J: *Interpretation of Diagnostic Tests*, 5th Edition. Boston, MA, Little, Brown, 1992. Used with permission.

interactions have altered desired levels of therapeutic drugs (Wallach 1992). Serum trough levels of mood stabilizers (such as lithium, valproate, or carbamazepine) and TCAs can be obtained to monitor therapeutic response in accordance with therapeutic levels for acute exacerbation and maintenance treatment of bipolar disorder.

Concomitant screening of blood tests before initiation of treatment with these mood stabilizers to assess for end-organ damage is also important. Follow-up screening tests during maintenance treatment is recommended at regular intervals, although the utility of these routine screens in detecting asymptomatic end-organ damage—such as an increase in liver function with valproate or renal impairment with lithium—is unclear. No clear consensus exists as to the appropriate interval for routine monitoring while a patient is taking a mood stabilizer, although most experts recommend screening every 3–6 months. However, some experts recommend that clinical monitoring of signs of toxicity may be more effective than periodic screening, as in the case of valproate and hepatotoxicity, when routine monitoring of liver function tests may have little predictive value (Marangell et al. 2002; Pellock and Willmore 1991). Listed in Table 4–4 are psychotropic medications for which therapeutic drug monitoring may be useful, as well as therapeutic and toxic drug levels and ancillary tests that should be monitored to prevent end-organ damage.

Similarly, drug levels of TCAs may also be obtained, although it is unclear whether blood levels of antidepressants correlate with therapeutic response. Four TCAs—imipramine, desipramine, amitriptyline, and nortriptyline—have been well studied, and generalizations can be made about the relationship of drug levels to therapeutic response. For imipramine, optimal response rates occur as blood levels reach 200–250 ng/mL, and levels greater than 250 ng/mL often produce more side effects but no change in antidepressant response (American Psychiatric Association Task Force 1985). On the other hand, nortriptyline appears to have a specific therapeutic window between 50 and 150 ng/mL, and poor clinical response occurs both above and below that window. Desipramine also appears to have a linear re-

Table 4–4. Medication monitoring

Medication type	Medication	Therapeutic range	Toxic level	Recommended screening
Mood stabilizer	Lithium	0.8–1.2 mEq/L	>1.5 mEq/L	Initiation: sodium, potassium, calcium, phosphate, BUN, creatinine, TSH, T_4, CBC, urinalysis, β-hCG if appropriate; ECG for patients over age 50 or with preexisting cardiac disease Maintenance: TSH, BUN/creatinine recommended every 6 months; ECGs as needed in patients over age 40 or with preexisting cardiac disease
	Valproate	50–150 μg/mL	>150 μg/mL	Initiation: CBC with platelets, LFTs; β-hCG if appropriate Maintenance: LFTs, CBC recommended every 6 months
	Carbamazepine	8–12 μg/mL	>12 μg/mL	Initiation: CBC with platelets, LFTs, BUN/creatinine Maintenance: CBC with platelets, LFTs, BUN/creatinine

Table 4–4. Medication monitoring *(continued)*

Medication type	Medication	Therapeutic range	Toxic level	Recommended screening
TCA	Imipramine + desipramine	125–250 ng/mL	>500 ng/mL or >1 g ingested	Desipramine is metabolite of imipramine Initiation: ECG in patients over age 40 or with preexisting cardiac disease for all TCAs
	Doxepin + metabolite desmethyl-doxepin	100–275 ng/mL	>500 ng/mL	Initiation: ECG in patients over age 40 or with preexisting cardiac disease for all TCAs
	Amitriptyline + nortriptyline	75–225 ng/mL	>500 ng/mL	Initiation: ECG in patients over age 40 or with preexisting cardiac disease for all TCAs
	Nortriptyline only	50–150 ng/mL	>50 ng/mL	Initiation: ECG in patients over age 40 or with preexisting cardiac disease for all TCAs
Antipsychotic	Olanzapine			Fasting serum glucose Triglycerides

Note. BUN=blood urea nitrogen; CBC=complete blood count; ECG=electrocardiogram; β-hCG=human chorionic gonadotropin beta; LFTs=liver function tests; T_4=thyroxine; TCA=tricyclic antidepressant; TSH=thyroid-stimulating hormone.

Source. Adapted from Wallach J: *Interpretation of Diagnostic Tests,* 5th Edition. Boston, MA, Little, Brown, 1992; and Hyman SE, Arana GW, Rosenbaum JF: *Handbook of Psychiatric Drug Therapy,* 3rd Edition. Boston, MA, Little, Brown, 1995. Used with permission.

lationship between drug concentration and clinical outcome, with plasma concentrations greater than 125 ng/mL significantly more effective than lower levels in depressed patients. Amitriptyline has been fairly well studied, although some studies have found a linear relationship similar to that of imipramine, whereas others have found a curvilinear relationship; still others have found no relationship at all between blood levels and clinical outcomes (American Psychiatric Association Task Force 1985). For the other TCAs that have been less well studied, drug levels can still be useful to confirm the presence of the drug or to confirm extremely high serum levels (Hyman et al. 1995).

Monitoring of blood levels of neuroleptics is not routinely used in clinical practice. Different methods for monitoring neuroleptic drugs have been developed, but a reliable therapeutic range has not been established, because there does not appear to be a consistent relationship between blood levels of neuroleptics and clinical response (Curry 1985). However, there are several clinical situations in which it may be useful to obtain blood levels of neuroleptics. Blood level monitoring may be useful to confirm the presence of the neuroleptic when adherence is a concern. It may be used to ascertain the presence of drug interactions in a patient who has relapsed or experienced an exacerbation of symptoms after a period of stabilization and has been taking drugs that may interact with neuroleptics, such as carbamazepine or fluoxetine. It may also be helpful to obtain drug levels in patients who develop excessive side effects to moderate doses of neuroleptics (Bernardo et al. 1993).

Diagnostic and laboratory monitoring is an important component of care for patients receiving neuroleptic medications. In patients who are over age 50 or who have preexisting cardiac disease, a screening ECG should be ordered before institution of antipsychotic medications, such as thioridazine or ziprasidone, that may cause prolongation of the QT_c interval (a marker for potentially life-threatening cardiac arrhythmias such as torsades de pointes). Follow-up ECGs should be ordered for any patient receiving treatment with antipsychotic medications should symptoms indicative of cardiac compromise appear. It is also recommended to perform screening laboratory studies at regular intervals to monitor glucose and metabolic dysregulation (hyperlipidemias, hypothyroidism) that is often associated with atypical antipsychotic medication.

Investigational Biological and Genetic Markers

There is considerable interest in isolating biological markers for neuropsychiatric illnesses for the purposes of improving the accuracy of psychiatric diagnoses, identifying patients at risk to prevent the development of the disorder, and predicting treatment response. Great strides have been made in discovering the genetic markers and pathophysiology underlying many primary neurological disorders, such as the dementias (Alzheimer's type and frontotemporal) and Huntington's disease. Sadly, no genetic or biological marker has yet been identified for any of the primary psychiatric disorders, although many studies are currently being undertaken. Table 4–5 lists some of the biomarkers being researched at this time.

Conclusion

Laboratory assessment is particularly important to the neuropsychiatric approach because of the complex array of neurological and medical illnesses that may underlie the psychiatric symptoms of the neuropsychiatric patient. Judicious choice of laboratory testing guided by a complete psychiatric assessment—including a thorough medical and psychiatric history, review of systems, and physical examination—may often uncover an unsuspected medical or neurological etiology underlying primarily psychiatric symptomatology. It is to be hoped that in the near future genetic and biological markers will be discovered and will attain a level of clinical utility so that a new and important dimension may be added to the uses of laboratory testing: the identification, biological treatment, and ultimately prevention of neuropsychiatric illnesses.

Table 4–5. Selected investigational biological and genetic markers

Type	Biomarker	Disease	Comments
Genetic markers	Chromosome 4p16.3	Huntington's disease	Trinucleotide (CAG) repeat
	Chromosome 4q21–22	Parkinson's disease	Some familial cases linked to mutation of the alpha-synuclein gene
	Chromosome 13	Wilson's disease	Copper transport gene
	Chromosome 21	Alzheimer's disease	Apolipoprotein E4 allele
	Chromosome 17q21–23	Frontotemporal dementias	Familial cases with mutations in the tau gene
	Chromosomes 18p, 18q, 21q, 12q, 4p	Bipolar disorder	Genetic linkages in families with bipolar disorder
Biochemical markers	CSF beta-amyloid$_{1-42}$	Alzheimer's disease	Reduced in CSF of patients with Alzheimer's disease compared with healthy elderly control subjects
	CSF tau	Alzheimer's disease	Elevated in CSF of patients with Alzheimer's disease compared with healthy control subjects
	CSF AD7C-NTP	Alzheimer's disease	
	CSF 14-3-3 protein	Creutzfeldt-Jacob disease	

Table 4–5. Selected investigational biological and genetic markers *(continued)*

Type	Biomarker	Disease	Comments
Catecholamines and metabolites	Dopamine Plasma homovanillic acid	Schizophrenia, depression	Decreases with antipsychotic treatment
	Norepinephrine 3-Methoxy-4-hydroxyphenylglycol	Major depression bipolar disorder	Low CSF levels associated with increased risk of suicidal behavior Urine levels may predict antidepressant response
Indoleamines and metabolites	Serotonin 5-Hydroxyindoleacetic acid	Depression, suicide, violence	Low CSF levels associated with suicidal behavior, aggression, impulsivity, depression, seizures, alcoholism High CSF levels associated with anxiety
Amino acids	Tryptophan Tyrosine Glycine Glutamate	Mood disorders	Low serum levels in depression Dietary neurotransmitter precursors being studied as treatment for depression

Table 4–5. Selected investigational biological and genetic markers *(continued)*

Type	Biomarker	Disease	Comments
Enzymes	Tyrosine hydroxylase Monoamine oxidase Dopamine beta-hydroxylase Adenyl cyclase Guanyl cyclase Nitric oxide synthase Catechol-*O*-methyltransferase	Mood and anxiety disorders, psychotic disorders	Numerous targets of antidepressant and mood stabilizer therapy
Psychoimmunological markers	Cytokine levels Immunoglobulin levels Viral titers	Depression	Proinflammatory cytokines are hypothesized to induce depression by their influence on the serotonergic, noradrenergic, and hypothalamic-pituitary-adrenal systems
Neuroendocrine markers	DST	Major depression	Limited clinical utility Posttreatment DST cortisol nonsuppression predictive of poor outcome and higher relapse risk

Table 4–5. Selected investigational biological and genetic markers *(continued)*

Type	Biomarker	Disease	Comments
	Thyrotropin-releasing hormone stimulation test	Major depression	Helpful in thyroid disorder diagnosis, but limited psychiatric utility Blunted response in up to 30% of depressed patients
Oculomotor measures	Smooth-pursuit eye movements Saccadic eye movements Visual fixation Pupillometry	Schizophrenia, neurodevelopmental disorders	Saccadic intrusions into smooth-pursuit eye movements are associated with schizophrenia

Note. CSF=cerebrospinal fluid; DST=dexamethasone suppression test.

Source. Adapted from Rosse RB, Deutsch LH, Deutsch SI: "Medical Assessment and Laboratory Testing in Psychiatry," in *Kaplan and Sadock's Comprehensive Textbook of Psychiatry*, 7th Edition, Volume 1. Edited by Sadock BJ, Sadock VA. Baltimore, MD, Lippincott Williams & Wilkins, 1999, pp. 732–754. Used with permission.

References

American Psychiatric Association Task Force on the Use of Laboratory Tests in Psychiatry: Tricyclic antidepressants—blood level measurements and clinical outcome: an APA Task Force report. Am J Psychiatry 142:155–162, 1985

Anfinson TJ, Kathol RG: Screening laboratory evaluation in psychiatric patients: a review. Gen Hosp Psychiatry 14(4):248–257, 1992

Anfinson TJ, Stoudemire A: Laboratory and neuroendocrine assessment in medical-psychiatric patients, in Psychiatric Care of the Medical Patient, 2nd Edition. Edited by Stoudemire A, Fogel BS, Greenberg DB. New York, Oxford University Press, 2000, pp 119–145

Barnes RF, Mason JC, Greer C, et al: Medical illness in chronic psychiatric outpatients. Gen Hosp Psychiatry 5(3):191–195, 1983

Bernardo M, Palao DJ, Arauxo A, et al: Monitoring plasma level of haloperidol in schizophrenia. Hosp Community Psychiatry 44(2):115–118, 1993

Brown M: An audit of the use of chest radiography in the elderly mentally ill. Int J Geriatr Psychiatry 10:155–158, 1995

Catalano G, Catalano MC, O'Dell KJ: The utility of laboratory screening in medically ill patients with psychiatric symptoms. Ann Clin Psychiatry 13(3):135–140, 2001

Curry SH: The strategy and value of neuroleptic drug monitoring. J Clin Psychopharmacol 5(5):263–271, 1985

Dolan JG, Mushlin AI: Routine laboratory testing for medical disorders in psychiatric inpatients. Arch Intern Med 145:2085–2088, 1985

Gomez-Gil E, Trilla A, Corbella B, et al: Lack of relevance of routine chest radiography in acute psychiatric admissions. Gen Hosp Psychiatry 24:110–113, 2002

Hall RCW, Popkin MK, Devaul RA, et al: Physical illness presenting as psychiatric disease. Arch Gen Psychiatry 35:1315–1320, 1978

Hall RCW, Gardner ER, Stickney SK, et al: Physical illness manifesting as psychiatric disease, II: analysis of a state hospital inpatient population. Arch Gen Psychiatry 37:989–995, 1980

Hall RCW, Gardner ER, Popkin MK, et al: Unrecognized physical illness prompting psychiatric admission: a prospective study. Am J Psychiatry 138:629–635, 1981

Hampton JR, Harrison MJ, Mitchell JR, et al: Relative contributions of history-taking, physical examination, and laboratory investigation to diagnosis and management of medical outpatients. BMJ 2:486–489, 1975

Harms HH, Hermans P: Admission laboratory testing in elderly psychiatric patients without organic mental syndromes: should it be routine? Int J Geriatr Psychiatry 9:133–140, 1994
Hollister LE: Electrocardiographic screening in psychiatric patients. J Clin Psychiatry 56:26–29, 1995
Honig A, Tan ES, Weenink A, et al: Utility of a symptom checklist for detecting physical disease in chronic psychiatric patients. Hosp Community Psychiatry 42:531–533, 1991
Hughes J, Barraclough BM: Value of routine chest radiography of psychiatric patients. Br Med J 281:1461–1462, 1980
Hyman SE, Arana GW, Rosenbaum JF: Handbook of Psychiatric Drug Therapy, 3rd Edition. Boston, MA, Little, Brown, 1995
Koran LM, Sox HC, Marton KI, et al: Medical evaluation of psychiatric patients. Arch Gen Psychiatry 46:733–740, 1989
Liston EH, Gerner RH, Robertson AG, et al: Routine thoracic radiography for psychiatric inpatients. Hosp Community Psychiatry 30:474–476, 1979
Marangell LB, Martinez JM, Silver JM, et al: Concise Guide to Psychopharmacology. Washington, DC, American Psychiatric Publishing, 2002
Mookhoek EJ, Sterrenburg-vdNieuwegiessen: Screening for somatic disease in elderly psychiatric patients. Gen Hosp Psychiatry 20:102–107, 1998
Olshaker JS, Browne B, Jarrard DA, et al: Medical clearance and screening of psychiatric patients in the emergency department. Acad Emerg Med 4:124–128, 1997
Pellock JM, Willmore LJ: A rational guide to routine blood monitoring in patients receiving antiepileptic drugs. Neurology 41:961–964, 1991
Sheline Y, Kehr C: Cost and utility of routine admission laboratory testing for psychiatric inpatients. Gen Hosp Psychiatry 12:329–334, 1990
Sox HC Jr, Koran LM, Sox CH, et al: A medical algorithm for detecting physical disease in psychiatric patients. Hosp Community Psychiatry 40:1270–1276, 1989
Wallach J: Interpretation of Diagnostic Tests, 5th Edition. Boston, MA, Little, Brown, 1992
White AJ, Barraclough B: Benefits and problems of routine laboratory investigations in adult psychiatric admissions. Br J Psychiatry 155:65–72, 1989
Willett AB, King T: Implementation of laboratory screening procedures on a short-term psychiatric inpatient unit. Dis Nerv Syst 38:867–870, 1977

Chapter 5

Selected Neuroimaging Topics in Psychiatric Disorders

Thomas E. Nordahl, M.D., Ph.D.
Ruth Salo, Ph.D.

Unlike most organs of the body, the brain has been less amenable to in vivo investigation until recent times. Researchers now have the capability to examine the fine structure and physiology of an intact brain in vivo with different imaging modalities. These imaging techniques have greatly increased the understanding of healthy brain function as well as the understanding of neuropsychiatric disorders. In this chapter we comment on selected neuroimaging findings in schizophrenia, major affective disorder, and obsessive-compulsive disorder (OCD). These disorders were chosen because there is a robust set of neuroimaging data available for review. We devote space to various uses of magnetic resonance imaging (MRI) and positron emission tomography (PET) for obtaining information about the brain as well as data related to pharmacological response. Studies of patient groups show that certain metabolic patterns increase the likelihood of response to treatment. However, imaging studies of an individual are currently not diagnostic and are not able to pre-

We thank Michael Buonocore, Robert Cohen, Chawki Benkelfat, and Edith V. Sullivan for their helpful comments on this chapter. We appreciate the help of Taka Natsuaki, Michael Buonocore, William Jagust, and Jamie Eberling, who provided images shown in this chapter.

dict response to pharmacological treatment. In the conclusion we discuss some of the future directions of MRI and PET as they relate to the pathophysiology of psychiatric disorders and their treatment.

Magnetic Resonance Imaging Techniques

During the nearly three decades since its inception, MRI has evolved considerably. In 1976 it was possible to acquire only a very blurry structural image. Currently with higher-field magnets and advanced pulse-sequence designs, it is possible to obtain high-resolution structural images of the brain or tissue of interest with submillimeter resolution. Such improved instrumentation allows for contrast between tissue types, allowing one to separate and segment brain tissue into gray matter, white matter, and cerebrospinal fluid. This permits the measurement of tissue volumes for the various brain structures in healthy and patient populations.

MRI is based on the phenomenon of nuclear magnetic resonance (NMR). NMR is the physical property whereby the nuclei of certain elements (such as hydrogen), when placed in a strong magnetic field and exposed to radio waves of a particular frequency, resonate or emit energy of the same frequency that can be detected as an NMR signal. This NMR signal can be localized in space by applying magnetic field gradients in three directions; subsequently, the localized signals can be converted to an image. Most MRI studies utilize the nuclei of hydrogen atoms (protons) as the source of the NMR signal. Basic MRI requires a strong primary magnetic field (B_0) that is parallel to the long axis of the tube-shaped device that a subject lies within. This large primary magnet generates these magnetic fields that align the hydrogen molecules (protons) within that field. The magnetic field gradient added to the main field allows one to select a slice for imaging. The radiofrequency pulses are applied perpendicularly to the main field at the same time as the gradient magnetic field, and these pulses perturb the aligned hydrogen molecules of the proscribed slice. These perturbed hydrogen molecules then precess about the axis of the primary magnetic field (B_0) and come back

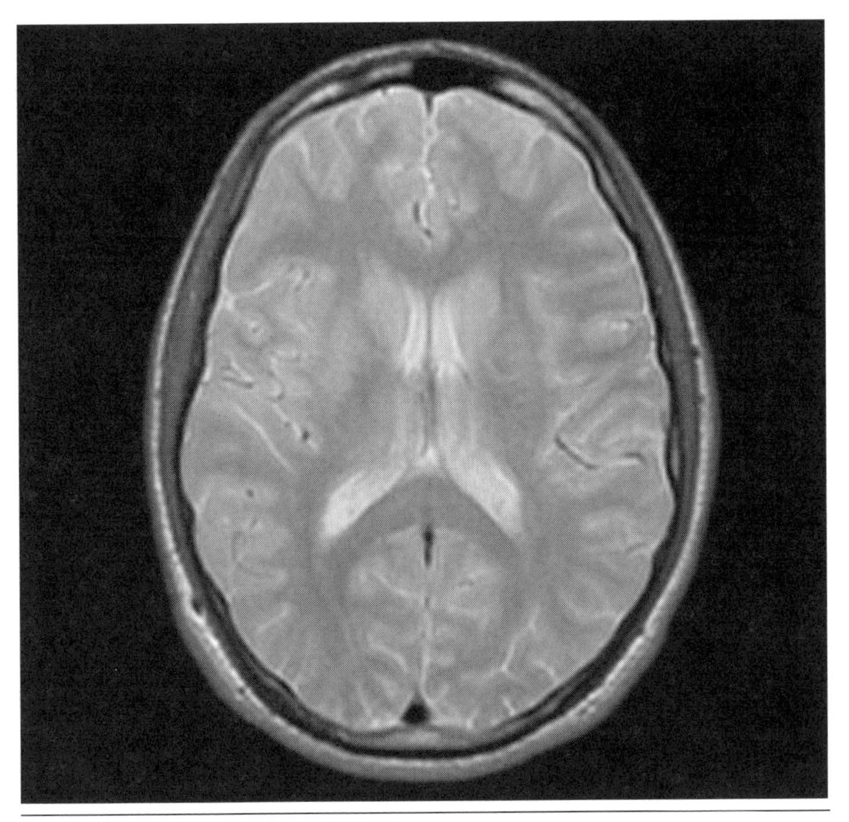

Figure 5–1. Proton-density magnetic resonance image.

to the initial alignment. The pattern of decay of the signal as the precessing protons come back into initial alignment gives information about the concentration of the signal source—the hydrogen atoms in water being imaged—and also reflects the chemical environment in which the signal source is found (Figure 5–1). Two characteristic relaxation times, T1 and T2, characterize the chemical environment (Figures 5–2 and 5–3).

In particular, MRI can determine whether the hydrogen atoms are present as free water or are partially bound in molecular structures found in fat, muscle, or blood. Differential patterns of radiofrequency and gradient pulse sequences can enhance certain tissue differences. The same ability to excite hydrogen nuclei in specific regions of the body has also been used to image blood flow. Thus, MRI can create images of blood flow similar to those

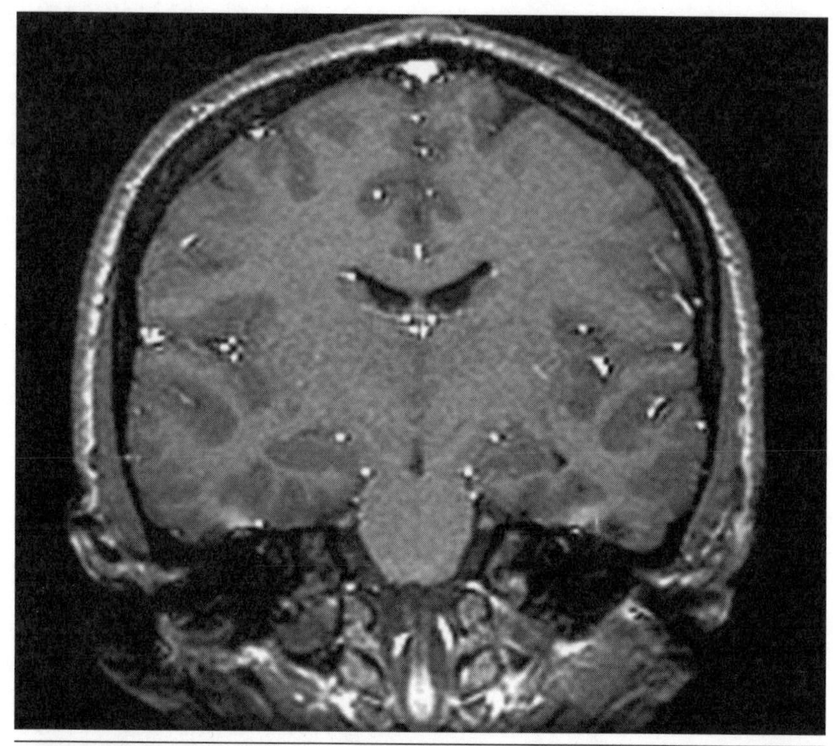

Figure 5–2. T1 magnetic resonance image.
T1 magnetic resonance image acquired in the coronal plane utilizing a spoiled gradient-echo sequence.

obtained by X-ray angiography but without injecting contrast media. These techniques can also be used to measure the direction and velocity of the flow. This approach is being utilized clinically in a wide range of cardiovascular studies (Dumoulin and Hart 1986).

Structural MRI Studies in Schizophrenia

In the past 25 years, significant work has been undertaken to understand the structure of the brain in individuals with schizophrenia. The majority of the structural imaging work in schizophrenia is currently performed with MRI. MRI has advantages over X-ray computed tomography (CT) in that images may be resliced in different angles; it has better ability to differentiate between gray matter, white matter, and cerebrospinal fluid; and it

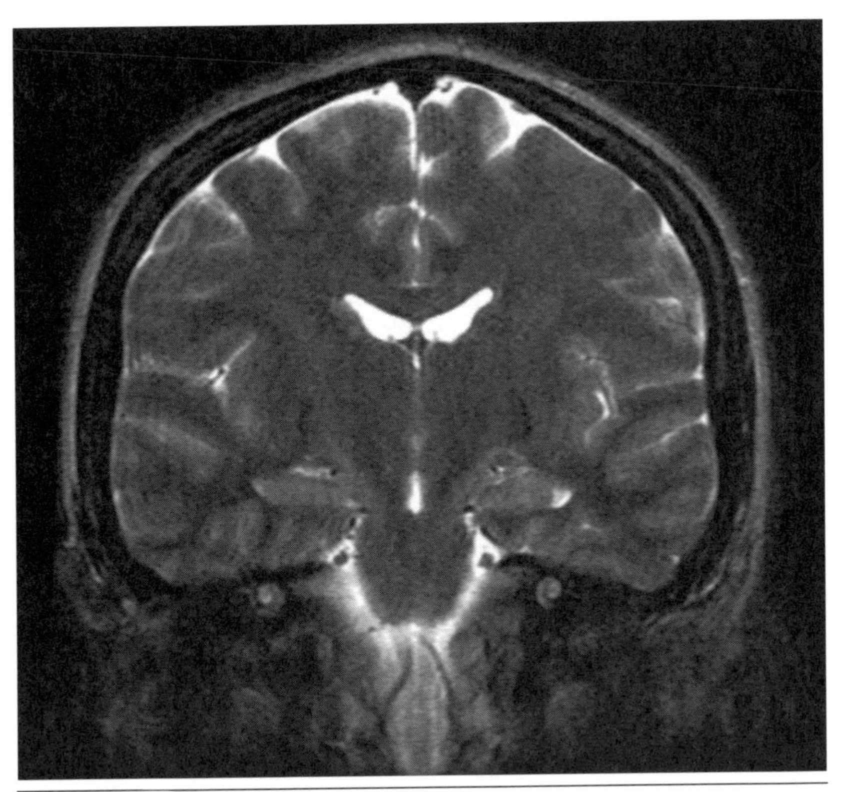

Figure 5–3. T2 magnetic resonance image.
T2 magnetic resonance image acquired in the coronal plane utilizing a fast spin echo sequence.

does not have the significant artifact problems near bony tissue that occur in X-ray CT. In a careful review of the MRI literature in schizophrenia, Shenton and colleagues (2001) examined 193 peer-reviewed MRI studies published between 1988 and August 2000. Of the studies reviewed, 80% reported ventricular enlargement, 74% reported a preferential involvement of medial temporal lobe structures, and 100% reported abnormalities in neocortical temporal lobe regions (superior temporal gyrus). Fifty-nine percent of the studies reviewed also reported moderate evidence for frontal lobe abnormalities, particularly prefrontal gray matter and orbitofrontal regions. Similarly, there was moderate evidence for parietal lobe abnormalities (60% of studies reviewed), particularly in the inferior parietal lobule. In addition, there was strong to moderate evidence for subcortical abnormalities (i.e., cavum septum pellucidum, 92% of studies reviewed; basal ganglia, 68% of studies reviewed; corpus callosum, 63% of studies reviewed; and thalamus, 42% of studies reviewed), with weaker evidence for cerebellar abnormalities (31% of studies reviewed) (Shenton et al. 2001).

Early Onset/Early in Course

Abnormalities have been found early in the course of the illness, with reports of enlarged lateral ventricles as well as cortical gray matter deficits in patients with first-episode schizophrenia (Lim et al. 1996). Giedd et al. (1999) studied children ages 14–16 with schizophrenia at baseline and then at a 2-year follow-up. They found striking progressive changes in brain volumes during adolescence for individuals with childhood-onset schizophrenia, with total cerebrum and hippocampal volume decreasing and lateral ventricular volume increasing with age. The developmental curves for these structures reached an asymptote by early adulthood for the childhood-onset group, whereas the researchers found development curves to be fairly constant during adolescence for the nonschizophrenic adolescents. An important issue in the imaging work is whether the abnormal changes over time are reflective of a neurodevelopmental disorder or a degenerative disorder. It is an issue that is difficult to settle, because pharmacological treatment has its own effects on structure and function. Changes in the volume of the putamen have been associated with pharmacological treatment with a typical antipsychotic medication (Corson et al. 1999). Patients with schizophrenia also abuse tobacco and other substances more than nonpsychotic control subjects, and these abuses may have their own effects on the brain. Examination of family members of a proband is potentially one way to control for the issues noted.

Magnetic Resonance Abnormalities of At-Risk Family Members of Patients With Schizophrenia

Sharma et al. (1999) examined cerebral hemispheric asymmetry in families in which several members were affected with schizophrenia compared with control subjects with no family history of schizophrenia. In contrast to the control subjects, who exhibited larger right than left prefrontal regions and larger left than right sensorimotor and occipitoparietal regions, the schizophrenic patients did not exhibit this normal brain asymmetry. The researchers noted that the presumed obligate carriers also did not exhibit asymmetries in these cortical regions, whereas the presumed nonobligate relatives showed lack of asymmetry only in the occipitoparietal region. The authors suggested that this lack of normal pattern of frontal and occipital asymmetry might be a marker for genetic liability for developing schizophrenia in families loaded for schizophrenia.

In related MRI work, Lawrie et al. (1999) studied 100 individuals at high risk of developing schizophrenia (two or more first-degree or second-degree relatives affected), 20 patients in their first episode of schizophrenia, and 30 healthy control subjects. These researchers found evidence of normal whole-brain volumes in the patients and in the high-risk group, but they found evidence of lower thalamic and hippocampal-amygdaloid complex volumes in the high-risk group compared with the control group. The authors suggested that their data might be helpful in screening individuals most likely to develop schizophrenia.

Structural MRI Studies in Obsessive-Compulsive Disorder

Unlike schizophrenia, in which the vast majority of structural volumetric studies reveal both cortical and subcortical abnormalities, the findings in OCD are less clear. Using structural MRI, Aylward et al. (1996) measured striatal and ventricular volume in 24 patients with OCD and 21 control subjects. In contrast to previously published studies, these researchers found no evidence of volume differences in striatal or ventricular regions between OCD patients and healthy control subjects. In a meta-analysis of OCD neuroimaging studies in unmedicated OCD patients using a variety of imaging techniques, no evidence of metabolic or perfusion abnormalities in the caudate nucleus was reported. We hasten to add that this does not rule out caudate nucleus pathology, because other imaging modalities have detected abnormalities in the caudate nucleus. This is discussed in more detail later (see "Magnetic Resonance Spectroscopy").

Structural MRI Studies in Major Depression

Multiple structural MRI studies have been performed in patients with unipolar and bipolar depression. Videbech (1997) performed a meta-analysis on the MRI studies in affective disorder, examining signal hyperintensities. He found abnormalities for frontal cortex and for basal ganglia in patients with unipolar and bipolar affective disorder. This would suggest a defective frontostriatal circuit. Elkis et al. (1995) performed a meta-analysis of studies of ventricular enlargement in multiple studies of patients with mood disorder (406 patients) and multiple studies of schizophrenia (599 patients). The researchers found the presence of ventricular enlargement and increased sulcal prominence in patients with affective disorder but not to the degree that was noted in patients with schizophrenia. We note that the mood disorder group was about 50% bipolar and 50% unipolar.

Functional MRI

Of greater interest to those who study cognitive processes is the discovery that MRI has the capability to extract information about the relative level of oxygenation of tissue. In studies of brain activation, changes in the oxygenation of hemoglobin are associated with external stimuli or cognitive challenge. It appears that hemoglobin changes between diamagnetic and paramagnetic states as a result of a relative change in oxygen extraction during sensory or cognitive challenge. Although this has become an immense field of research, a complete discussion of it is beyond the scope of this chapter. Interested readers are referred to existing surveys of this burgeoning field (Cabeza and Nyberg 2000).

Magnetic Resonance Spectroscopy

Magnetic resonance spectroscopy (MRS) is a valuable tool to examine the presence of neuronal damage or deterioration in psychiatric disorders. MRS is based on the same NMR principles as MRI and produces patterns of signals, or spectra, that allow visualization of neurochemicals in vivo. The individual peaks in the spectrum represent information about the chemical makeup of the tissue under examination, with changes in these spectra over time following the changes in concentrations of biological compounds. MRS allows for the visualization of a diverse group of markers of cellular integrity and function, including those of living neurons (*N*-acetylaspartate [NAA]), high-energy metabolic products (creatine), cell membrane synthesis or degradation (choline), and glia (myo-inositol). NAA is believed to be present almost exclusively in neurons and their dendritic and axonal processes (Tsai and Coyle 1995). In a number of clinical diseases associated with neuronal damage or loss, lower NAA concentrations in specific regions have been demonstrated on proton spectroscopy. Examples include Alzheimer's disease (Pfefferbaum et al. 1999), seizure disorder (Ende et al. 1997), multiple sclerosis (Gonen et al. 2000), human immunodeficiency virus–associated brain disease (Chang et al. 1995), alcoholism (Schweinsburg et al. 2001), brain infarction (Bruhn et al. 1989), and head trauma (Friedman et al. 1999).

Although structural MRI employs hydrogen protons almost exclusively, MRS uses a number of elements, including hydrogen (proton), phosphorus 31, fluorine 15, lithium 7, sodium 23, and carbon 13. Compared with MRI, MRS requires that a relatively large volume be sampled so that a sufficient signal can be obtained. MRS has a volume resolution of about 1 cc from H 1 or proton spectroscopy of metabolites, whereas a volume of 6 cc or more is necessary for phosphorus spectroscopy. These are large volumes compared with the resolution for MRI, which measures the concentrated protons in water. Despite these limitations, MRS has made significant contributions to the imaging of biological function.

Two MRS techniques are available in proton spectroscopy: single-voxel proton MRS, in which a preselected region of interest is sampled, and proton magnetic resonance spectroscopic imaging (MRSI), in which several brain regions can be sampled simultaneously and multiple spectra can be obtained (Figure 5–4).

Although single-voxel techniques may yield greater signal-to-noise ratios, MRSI possesses the ability to better define neurochemical differences between brain regions. Because of this, MRSI is currently used extensively for diagnostic purposes in clinical settings. MRS has made significant contributions to the understanding of neurochemical function to date and has great potential to contribute to the further understanding of neurochemical differences associated with neuropsychiatric disorders and for observing neurochemical changes over time (Adalsteinsson et al. 2000).

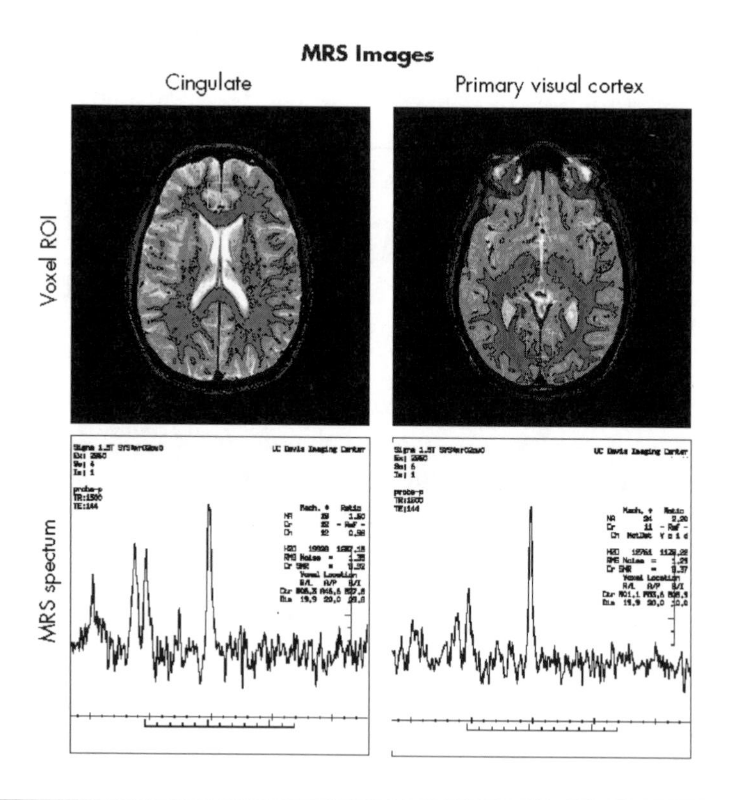

Figure 5–4. Proton magnetic resonance spectroscopic images and associated spectra.

Two regions of interest (ROIs) (anterior cingulum and primary visual cortex) are studied. The *upper image* represents the location of the magnetic resonance spectroscopy (MRS) voxel superimposed on the corresponding fast spin echo proton-density image. The *lower portion* of the figure is the MRS spectrum of the respective voxel.

MRS Studies in Schizophrenia

Temporal Cortical Regions

The most consistent MRS findings in patients with schizophrenia have emerged in medial temporal lobe regions, with most studies (but not all) reporting abnormally low NAA values within medial temporal regions (Bertolino et al. 1998; Deicken et al. 1998; Nasrallah et al. 1994; Yurgelun-Todd et al. 1996). Using MRSI techniques to measure levels of NAA, creatine, and choline, Deicken et al. (1998) found that relative to the control group, the patients demonstrated significantly lower NAA concentration bilaterally in hippocampal regions, with no group differences in choline noted. Some studies have reported greater right than left temporal lobe NAA abnormalities in patients with schizophrenia (Nasrallah et al. 1994), whereas others have found no differences in NAA levels between schizophrenic patients and healthy control subjects (Bartha et al. 1999; Buckley et al. 1994).

Frontal Brain Regions

Several studies have reported lower NAA concentrations within the frontal lobes of schizophrenia patients compared with control subjects (Bertolino et al. 1998; Buckley et al. 1994; Cecil et al. 1999; Deicken et al. 1997a). Deicken and colleagues (1997a) found that relative to a comparison group, schizophrenic patients demonstrated significantly lower levels of NAA, and no correlation emerged between NAA concentration and duration of illness or medication dosage. No differences between groups or lateralized asymmetries in choline or creatine were noted. Studies conducted in children with schizophrenia-spectrum disorder have reported similar patterns of abnormally low frontal NAA concentration (Brooks et al. 1998), suggesting that abnormalities in frontal NAA level are present in both early-onset and late-onset schizophrenia. Other researchers have also suggested that MRS abnormalities noted in the frontal and temporal cortices of the brain in schizophrenia may be more prevalent in white matter than in gray matter (Bartha et al. 1999; Lim et al. 1998; Yurgelun-Todd et al. 1996).

Pharmacological Effects

MRS may be an ideal tool to investigate brain changes due to antipsychotic treatment at the neuronal level. Using MRS, Bertolino et al. (2001) employed a within-subjects design in which 23 schizophrenia patients were studied twice (once while the patients were taking medication and again 2 weeks after discontinuation of medication). Levels of NAA were measured in several regions, including frontal and hippocampal areas. Increases in NAA concentration were noted solely in the frontal region as a function of neuroleptic treatment. It should be noted that in this study 10 of the patients were taking typical neuroleptics and the remaining 13 were taking atypical neuroleptics, most notably clozapine and risperidone. A pair of studies directly compared the effects of haloperidol and clozapine on the levels of the metabolites NAA, choline, and creatine within the basal ganglia, anterior cingulate cortex, and frontal regions (Braus et al. 2002; Bustillo et al. 2001). Patients treated with atypical antipsychotics exhibited higher NAA concentrations than those treated with typical antipsychotics. In contrast, Deicken et al. (1997b) found no difference in NAA levels in the anterior cingulate cortex as a function of medication type. Discrepancies in the findings may be due to a number of methodological differences such as size of the regions sampled, absolute levels versus ratios of metabolites measured, and correction for cerebrospinal fluid volume. Further research is needed so that the effects of antipsychotic medication on NAA levels in the human brain can be better understood.

Symptom Correlates

MRS techniques have great potential to elucidate the interaction between neuronal changes and clinical symptomatology. Correlations between lower NAA levels and higher psychotic symptoms have been noted in patients with schizophrenia, suggesting that altered function of the frontal lobe may contribute to greater positive symptomatology (Bertolino et al. 1999; Deicken et al. 1994). Combining single-photon emission computed tomography and MRS techniques, Bertolino et al. (1999) found an inverse correlation between NAA levels within the prefrontal cortex and striatal dopamine D_2 receptor availability, suggesting that abnormal neuronal integrity within the prefrontal cortex may contribute to greater dopamine release in the striatum.

In a study by Deicken et al. (1994), in vivo phosphorus 31 MRSI was performed on 20 patients with chronic schizophrenia and 16 nonschizophrenic control subjects to determine if there were specific changes in high-energy phosphorus and phospholipid metabolism in the frontal lobes of schizophrenic patients. Patients with schizophrenia exhibited higher phosphodiesters and lower phosphocreatine levels in both the left and right frontal regions, which in turn correlated with severity of psychiatric symptomatology as assessed by the Brief Psychiatric Rating Scale.

MRS Studies in Obsessive-Compulsive Disorder

Results from MRI volumetric studies of subjects with OCD have yielded inconsistent results. MRS may prove to be a more sensitive measure to elucidate the neural abnormalities associated with OCD. It has been suggested that disruptions in the basal ganglia–thalamic–cortical circuit may underlie the pathology of OCD. Consistent with this view, abnormally low levels of NAA have been observed within the caudate nucleus in the absence of volumetric changes (Bartha et al. 1998; Ebert et al. 1997). Additional studies have also reported abnormally low medial thalamic NAA/choline ratios in a sample of pediatric outpatients with a diagnosis of OCD. These early findings of regional abnormalities as noted by MRS in the absence of volumetric differences within the same regions suggest that reductions in NAA concentration may occur before the detection of neuronal loss by more traditional MRI methods. Therefore, the application of MRS to OCD and other psychiatric disorders may offer an early window into pathological changes in the brain.

MRS Studies in Depression

Although studies of affective disorders using proton MRS and phosphorus 31 MRS are still in an early stage, several patterns have nonetheless emerged: 1) higher choline peaks in basal ganglia regions, 2) lower phosphomonoester levels in frontal regions, and 3) higher phosphodiester levels in frontal regions of patients with unipolar depression than in control subjects. Abnormally high levels of choline have been reported in both older (Charles et al. 1994) and younger (Renshaw et al. 2001) depressed patients. Certain MRS findings are more predictive of a clinical response to antidepressant treatment. Renshaw et al. (2001) examined certain purines in patients with major depression utilizing both proton MRS and phosphorus 31 MRS. They found no overall differences in purine resonance intensities between the depressed patients at baseline and the control subjects. However, the researchers also found that female depressed patients who responded to treatment had a 30% lower purine level than did female patients who did not respond to subsequent fluoxetine treatment. The authors note that beyond predictive value for women, the MRS data suggest that agents that increase levels of brain purine, such as adenosine, may have antidepressant efficacy.

Diffusion Tensor Imaging

Diffusion tensor imaging (DTI) has emerged as a powerful, noninvasive imaging tool that gives a measure of the pattern of connectivity between neural structures by examining the restricted flow patterns of water molecules in axonal pathways and white matter substrates. When water molecules are flowing randomly in cerebrospinal fluid or cortical gray matter, the environment is said to be isotropic. In contrast, when the environment is constrained by white matter cell membranes (i.e., organelles and axonal bundles), the diffusion is restricted such that flow is greater along the axon than perpendicular to it. This diffusion or flow pattern is called anisotropy. DTI techniques are necessary to measure the directional flow of water molecules in anisotropic environments by combining a number of diffusion-weighed images along with a baseline or reference image to characterize the flow of water molecules in three-dimensional space (Figure 5–5). Different measures can be obtained from the DTI images, such as fractional anisotropy (FA) and coherence (C) indices. FA is computed on a voxel-to-voxel basis and reflects the degree or fraction of the total anisotropic tensor (Figure 5–6). FA values vary across regions and tissue types. Regions where fibers are organized in parallel, such as the corpus callosum, have high FA values approaching 1, whereas FA values in the ventricular cerebrospinal fluid are closer to 0, reflecting a random or isotropic diffusion pattern (Pierpaoli and Basser 1996). C represents the coherence between voxels in the white matter (Pfefferbaum et al. 2000). DTI techniques are extremely valuable when examining axonal integrity and connectivity of brain structures and have important applications to the study of neuropsychiatric disorders.

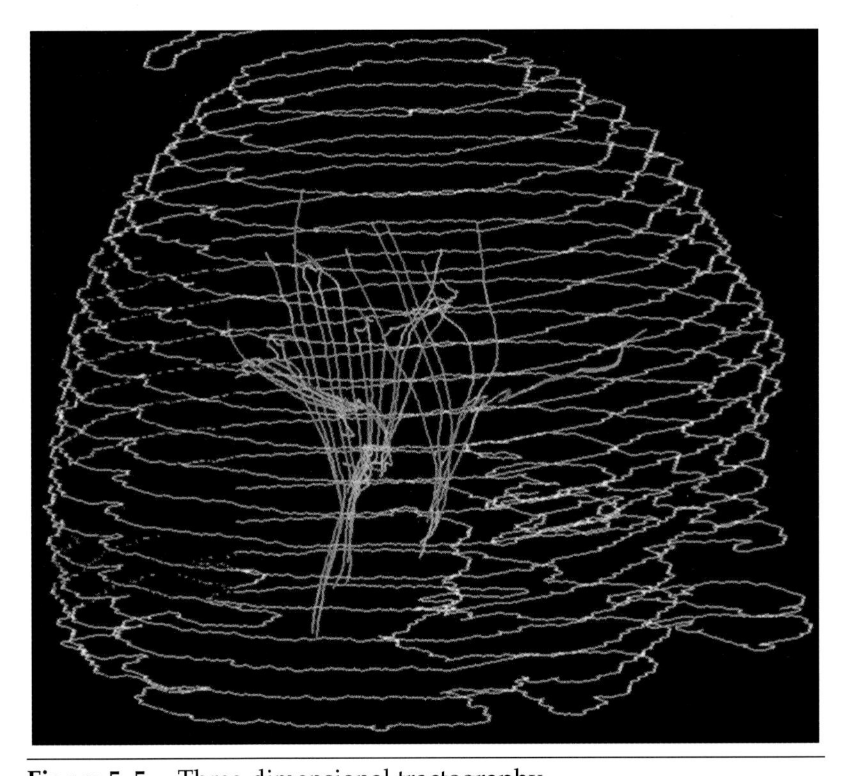

Figure 5–5. Three-dimensional tractography.
Using special magnetic resonance imaging sequences to measure the diffusion of water in all directions, the resulting diffusion-weighted images can be processed further to reveal the direction of the white-matter nerve tracts. The *color lines* represent the paths of the corticospinal tracts. (Image courtesy of Michael Buonocore.)

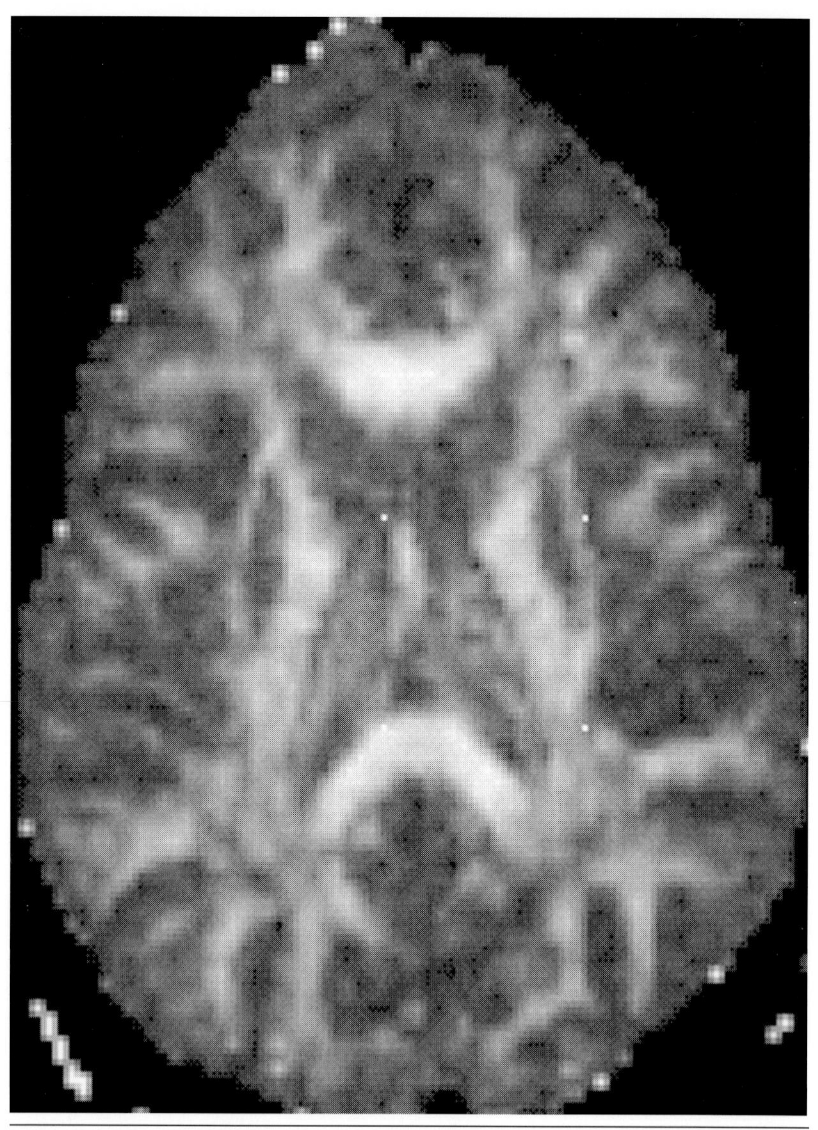

Figure 5–6. Fractional anisotropy image.

DTI Studies in Schizophrenia

Many researchers have proposed a disconnection syndrome to account for many of the core symptoms associated with schizophrenia. This theory suggests that neural connectivity may be abnormal in patients with schizophrenia as a result of altered synaptogenesis or abnormal dendritic pruning during development (Feinberg 1990). White matter abnormalities have also been detected in schizophrenia, with lowered markers of neuronal integrity having been observed in the frontal white matter of patients with schizophrenia (Lim et al. 1998). Although volumetric measurements of white matter macrostructure can be obtained through traditional MRI techniques, currently DTI is the only in vivo tool capable of measuring white matter microstructure within the human brain. To date only a handful of DTI studies have been conducted in patients with schizophrenia; the results are reviewed below.

In a study by Lim et al. (1999), FA was measured in 10 patients with schizophrenia and 10 matched control subjects. The researchers found widespread abnormally low FA values in the schizophrenia patients ranging from the frontal cortex bilaterally all the way back to the posterior visual cortex. In a subsequent study, Foong et al. (2002) obtained FA measures within the corpus callosum (genu and splenium) of 20 patients with schizophrenia and 20 control subjects. Differences in FA values were noted, with schizophrenia patients exhibiting lower FA values within the splenium compared with control subjects. Buchsbaum et al. (1998) conducted a study that employed both DTI and PET. In addition to reductions in FA values within the prefrontal cortex in 5 schizophrenia patients, the researchers also reported significantly lower correlation coefficients between prefrontal and striatal metabolism in the schizophrenia patients compared with control subjects. The authors interpreted these convergent findings to represent abnormally low frontal-striatal connectivity in schizophrenia. Steel et al. (2001) also examined prefrontal regions in schizophrenia patients and control subjects. In contrast to the findings of Buchsbaum et al. (1998), these researchers did not find frontal white matter FA differences between groups, although they did note other abnormalities.

In a recent DTI study Kubicki et al. (2002) examined white matter microstructure in the uncinate fasciculus, a prominent white matter tract connecting the frontal and temporal cortices, in 15 schizophrenia patients and 18 control subjects. The findings revealed that the normal left-greater-than-right FA asymmetry in this area, present in the control subjects, was absent in the schizophrenia patients. The authors interpreted this lack of normal asymmetry as a possible marker of disrupted connectivity. One study linking psychiatric symptomatology and DTI measurements has also been conducted. Wolkin et al. (2003) found that lower FA values in the inferior frontal white matter correlated with greater negative symptoms in patients with schizophrenia.

DTI Studies in Depression

Only two studies of depression using DTI techniques have been published, and both of these studies were carried out in geriatric populations (Alexopoulos et al. 2002; Taylor et al. 2001). Alexopoulos and colleagues (2002) tested a group of 13 older individuals (age range, 60–77 years) who met criteria for major depression. All 13 subjects were treated with citalopram. Five subjects remained depressed, with the other 8 showing signs of remission according to DSM-IV criteria (American Psychiatric Association 1994). All of the subjects underwent MRI scans on which DTI analyses were carried out. The results showed lower FA values bilaterally in dorsolateral prefrontal regions (10–15 mm above the anterior commissure–posterior commissure plane) correlated with low response rates. No such relationship was observed in inferior frontal or temporal cortical regions. The authors interpreted these findings as possible evidence of disconnectivity between dorsal frontal and limbic structures that may be related to treatment response in depression.

DTI has enormous potential for the examination of microstructural white matter changes in the psychiatric population. It is only a matter of time before this technique is applied to a wider range of psychiatric illnesses, including bipolar disorder and anxiety disorders; it is also sure to be used more extensively in substance abuse.

Positron Emission Tomography

PET has evolved significantly during the past quarter of a century. PET provides physiological information about the tissue being sampled via the detection of paired 511-keV photons that are emitted by radioactive decay. By detecting the simultaneous arrival of these photons at crystal sensors, the electronics determine the line path (chord) on which the isotope existed at the time that the radioactive decay occurred. The PET study requires 1) a PET camera with sensors that pick up (simultaneous) pairs of photons emanating from tissue being sampled, 2) a compound labeled with a positron emitter, and 3) a compartmental model characterizing relevant physiological processes that the radiolabeled compound undergoes. Positron emitters release a positron when a proton is converted to a neutron. This released positron then annihilates an electron, resulting in the emission of two gamma ray photons at a 180-degree eccentricity to each other. Numerous elements have positron-emitting isotopes, including several commonly found in biological molecules, for example, fluorine 18, carbon 11, oxygen 15, and nitrogen 13. The acquired imaging data as well as the compartmental model are then utilized to obtain the physiological rates of the biological processes being sampled.

The radioligand [^{18}F]-2-fluoro-D-deoxyglucose (FDG) is used most frequently in PET studies. FDG PET permits the calculation of average glucose metabolic rate per volume and is utilized clinically as well as in neuropsychiatric research (Figure 5–7). Clinically, an FDG PET study can distinguish the metabolically active periphery of a tumor from its necrotic core, thus serving as an indicator of the effectiveness of chemical or radiation therapy (Valk and Dillon 1991). The application of PET to neuropsychiatry includes the imaging of neuroreceptors, neurotransmitter kinetics, transporters, and blood flow and the measurement of regional glucose metabolism (see Patterson and Kotrla 2002 for a sample list of radioligands). Regional glucose metabolic and regional blood flow studies generally produce data that have been normalized in some fashion, for example, to average whole brain function. This is done in large part to increase the likelihood of observing the typically subtle abnormalities observed in psychiatric disorders.

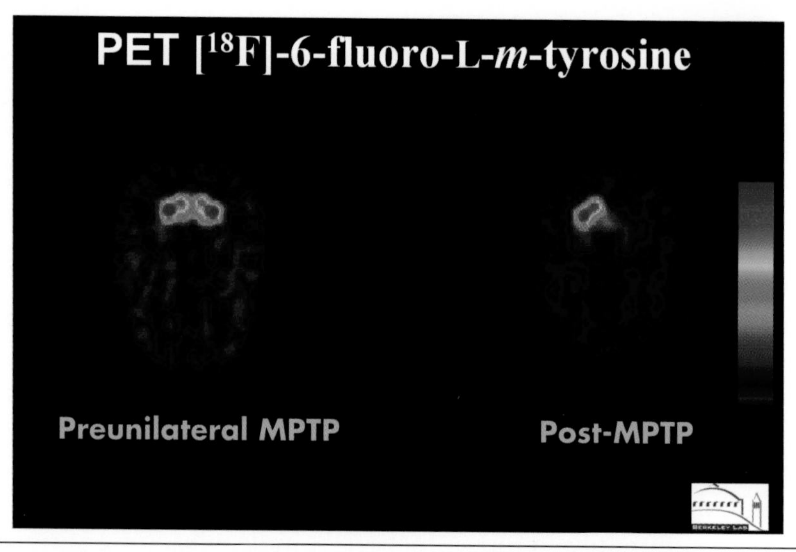

Figure 5–7. Positron emission tomographic dopamine image.
Animal studies have contributed important information regarding dopamine function. Utilizing positron emission tomography (PET) and radioligand fluorometa-tyrosine F 18, the effects of unilateral application of 1-methyl-4-phenyl-1,2,3,6-tetrahydropyridine (MPTP) on striatal dopa decarboxylase activity are examined in monkey brain. (Images courtesy of Jamie Eberling and William Jagust.)

PET Studies in Schizophrenia

Many PET studies of patients with schizophrenia have produced evidence of relative hypometabolism or hypofrontality in the prefrontal cortex (Buchsbaum et al. 1982; Ingvar and Franzen 1974; Wolkin et al. 1985). The studies in which hypofrontality was reported have typically involved patients with chronic schizophrenia who required extensive neuroleptic treatment and lengthy periods of hospitalization. Findings of hypofrontality are also more common in samples of patients with prominent negative symptoms (Tamminga et al. 1992; Wolkin et al. 1985), as opposed to higher-functioning patients (Gur et al. 1995; Volkow et al. 1986). Most studies—whether of high-functioning or of low-functioning patients—found limbic metabolic abnormalities, such as in the temporal lobe or the anterior cingulum (Nordahl et al. 2001; Tamminga et al. 1992).

Certain baseline FDG PET findings have been found to be predictive of a positive clinical response. In a study of schizophrenia patients who had been withdrawn from medication, Buchsbaum et al. (1992) noted that patients who exhibited lower glucose metabolic rates in the basal ganglia were more likely to respond after antipsychotic medication was restarted than were patients who had elevated basal ganglia metabolism at baseline. Using FDG PET, Cohen et al. (1998) examined 19 male medication-withdrawn schizophrenia patients and 41 control subjects while they were performing an auditory sustained-attention task during tracer uptake. The researchers observed that some patients exhibited lower right midprefrontal metabolism independent of task performance, which in turn predicted better clinical response. In contrast, high basal ganglia metabolic rates and low mid–cingulate cortex metabolism predicted poor treatment response. The authors concluded that the sustained attention pathway and its distributed network of brain structures are likely to play an important role in the expression of psychotic symptoms and the mediation of their response to antipsychotic medication.

Receptor/Transporter Findings in Schizophrenia

The development of PET has now made it feasible to study radioligand binding to receptors in the living human brain (Wagner et al. 1983). After intravenous injection of a radioligand, the PET camera system measures regional brain radioactivity as a function of time. Because of their importance in the treatment response in schizophrenia, dopamine D_2 receptors were among the first targeted for study. Raclopride, a highly selective D_2 receptor antagonist, has been labeled with the positron-emitting isotope carbon 11 for use in PET examination of central dopamine D_2 receptors in humans (Farde et al. 1989). Equilibrium is rapidly established after ligand injection, allowing the determination of estimates of receptor density and binding affinity.

Interpretation of studies of D_2 receptor binding in schizophrenia has been problematic, with some studies finding a greater number of striatal dopamine D_2 receptors in schizophrenia and others reporting no difference. Seeman et al. (1987) found a bimodal distribution of D_2 receptor densities in postmortem striatal tissue, with modes at 14 and 26 pmol/g. The authors believed that the higher values could not be fully explained by neuroleptic treatment before death. In vivo PET studies—primarily from Europe, such as that by Hietala et al. (1994)—have not shown any significant difference in striatal D_2 receptor density or binding affinity between neuroleptic-naïve patients and healthy control subjects. However, Hietala et al. (1994) noted that 4 of their 13 drug-naïve patients had relatively high receptor density values, and 2 patients had values as high as double the mean control value. The story remains open, and to some extent this may be because of the heterogeneity of the disorder. Studying patients who have similar biological or genetic markers may yield more consistent results. The subset of patients with prominent elevations in D_2 receptor densities before antipsychotic treatment may be differentially responsive to treatment or may have greater risk for motoric side effects than patients with essentially normal densities of D_2 receptors before treatment.

Another interesting body of research suggests that although schizophrenia patients might not have abnormal baseline receptor levels or abnormal dopamine levels, they may have a greater response to amphetamine challenge, releasing more dopamine than would be seen in control subjects (Breier et al. 1997; Laruelle et al. 1996). Using PET and the tracer raclopride C 11, researchers reported that the relative amount of dopamine released per subject group was based on the change in striatal D_2 receptor sites available to the PET ligand after the acute amphetamine challenge. Further studies need to be performed that control for the degree of tobacco use or even stress around the time of the PET study. It has been reported that elements other than nicotine in tobacco smoke inhibit monoamine oxidase function, and this fact could allow more dopamine to remain in the synapse and compete with the PET ligand for binding sites in smokers (Fowler et al. 1996a, 1996b). As is known, most patients with schizophrenia smoke tobacco (de Leon et al. 2002).

Treatment of schizophrenia primarily involves D_2 antagonism but not D_1 antagonism. Utilizing PET and the tracers SCH23390 C 11 for D_1 receptors and raclopride C 11 for D_2 receptors, Farde et al. (1989) determined striatal dopamine receptor occupancy in schizophrenic patients treated with clinical doses of conventional and atypical antipsychotics. The researchers found that long-term treatment with conventional or typical antipsychotic medications led to D_2 receptor binding greater than 64%, but that fewer than 36% of D_1 receptors were occupied, with no binding occurring in some cases. However, the patients receiving clozapine treatment had lower D_2 receptor occupancy (between 40% and 65%) but higher D_1 receptor binding (e.g., 42%) than with the typical antipsychotic medications. The dopamine D_1 system is less likely to play a role in the clinical response to typical antipsychotic medications, but it might play a role in the response to clozapine.

The receptor occupancy curves as a function of clinical dose permit estimation of the clinical antipsychotic doses that would be sufficient to achieve a certain degree of D_2 binding. For example, treatment with 4–12 mg of haloperidol led to D_2 receptor binding ranging from 81% to 89%.

Researchers have attempted to understand what accounts for the clinical differences between the typical antipsychotic medications (e.g., haloperidol and fluphenazine) and the atypical antipsychotics (e.g., clozapine, olanzapine, risperidone, and ziprasidone). In contrast to most typical antipsychotic medications, the so-called atypical antipsychotic agents have relatively greater 5-hydroxytryptamine type 2 (5-HT_2) antagonism than dopamine D_2 antagonism. Using PET, Farde et al. (1995) examined D_2 and 5-HT_2 receptor binding in risperidone-treated patients with schizophrenia and contrasted the binding with the receptor binding they had previously found in neuroleptic-naïve patients. After 4 weeks of treatment with 6 mg/day of risperidone, the D_2 receptor occupancy in the striatum measured with radiolabeled raclopride was 75%–80%, whereas the 5-HT receptor occupancy in the frontal cortex measured with labeled *N*-methyl spiperone was 78%–88%. This pattern of greater 5-HT_2 binding than D_2 binding with risperidone is a pattern that has been noted for the other atypical antipsychotic medications (e.g., clozapine, quetiapine, and olanzapine). Some have suggested that this relative pattern of binding (5-HT_2 > D_2) might account for better treatment response, especially with negative symptoms, or may account for the lower degree of motoric side effects seen with these treatments (Meltzer et al. 1989).

Kapur and Seeman (2001) wrote an insightful review of the binding patterns of the typical and atypical antipsychotic medications. They reviewed a large number of treatment studies encompassing 7,000 patients. In the article the authors challenged the theory discussed above that proposes that relatively high 5-HT_2 receptor occupancy may be associated with the atypical effect. They also noted that most studies of atypical antipsychotic medications report lower extrapyramidal side effects and lower prolactin levels but consistently find lower rates of negative symptoms. The authors claim that the reduction in motoric side effects is primarily due to decreased binding of the D_2 receptors and that this lower binding is the result of a faster rate of dissociation of the antipsychotic medication from the D_2 receptor. The argument is that if the D_2 occupancy rate is excessive, atypicality is lost even in the presence of high 5-HT_2 occupancy. In support of this last argument, Kapur and Seeman note that high 5-HT_2 receptor binding is also seen with many typical antipsychotic medications, yet motoric side effects commonly occur. They further note that binding to 65% or more of D_2 receptors produces antipsychotic effects, whereas binding to more than 78% of receptors leads to extrapyramidal side effects.

PET Studies in Obsessive-Compulsive Disorder

OCD is a severe anxiety disorder that responds clinically to selective serotonin reuptake inhibitors (SSRIs) but not to noradrenergic or dopamine reuptake inhibitors. Functional imaging techniques have implicated (orbital) frontal-subcortical networks in the pathophysiology of OCD. In particular, many FDG PET studies have found abnormally high glucose metabolism in the orbitofrontal cortex (Baxter et al. 1987; Nordahl et al. 1989) and anterior cingulum (Perani et al. 1995; Swedo et al. 1989).

Successful pharmacological treatment of OCD has been associated with significantly decreased metabolism in the orbitofrontal cortex (as measured by PET) (Benkelfat et al. 1990), anterior cingulate cortex (Perani et al. 1995; Swedo et al. 1992), and caudate nucleus (Baxter et al. 1992; Benkelfat et al. 1990). Furthermore, Baxter et al. (1992) reported that significant decreases in caudate nucleus metabolism after behavioral therapy compared with the baseline study were similar to those observed after treatment with fluoxetine. Benkelfat et al. (1990) and others (Baxter et al. 1992) observed that when comparing OCD patients who responded with those who did not respond, only the responders showed significant decrease in caudate nucleus metabolism after treatment. We contrast baseline metabolic response predictions in depressed patients with those of OCD patients under "PET Studies in Depression" below.

PET Studies in Depression

There is an extensive body of literature on regional cerebral glucose metabolic and flow abnormalities in depression. Many lines of evidence have implicated frontal, striatal, and limbic structures in the pathophysiology of depression (see reviews by Brody et al. 2001; Ketter et al. 1996; Rogers et al. 1998). Abnormalities have typically involved abnormally low metabolic function in limbic and dorsolateral prefrontal cortical regions, whereas potentially abnormally high metabolic rates may be found in the ventrolateral frontal cortex. Certain baseline metabolic patterns are predictive of positive clinical response to treatment. Mayberg et al. (1997) found that baseline glucose metabolism in the anterior cingulate cortex predicted response to antidepressant medication in patients with unipolar depression. The patients who responded exhibited higher pretreatment glucose metabolism in a rostral region of the anterior cingulum (Brodmann's areas 24a and 24b) than did both nonresponders and control subjects. This is in apparent contradiction to other baseline studies that have reported abnormally low anterior cingulate cortex metabolism in patients with major depression. However, the studies reporting anterior cingulate cortex hypometabolism in depression typically sampled the dorsal anterior cingulum (Brodmann's area 32).

To clarify whether different networks of brain regions were involved in the prediction of treatment response in OCD and major depression, Saxena and colleagues (2003) directly investigated this issue by testing 27 patients solely with depression, 27 patients solely with OCD, and 17 patients with both OCD and major depression. They obtained a baseline FDG PET study in these patients, who were without psychotropic medications for a minimum of 4 weeks, and then a follow-up study after the patients had been treated clinically with 30–60 mg of paroxetine. The authors found that improvement in OCD symptoms was significantly correlated with higher pretreatment glucose metabolism in the right caudate nucleus (partial r=–0.53), whereas improvement in symptoms of major depression disorder was significantly correlated with lower pretreatment metabolism in the amygdala (partial r=0.71) and thalamus (partial r=0.34) and with higher pretreatment metabolism in the medial prefrontal cortex and the rostral anterior cingulate gyrus. These are very interesting findings, because this study utilized the same pharmacological treatment and imaging procedure for patients with both disorders. A different neural network may be involved in treatment response for the two disorders. It is important to remember that these studies examined group means of those who responded as well as those who did not respond. Researchers have been unable to predict the clinical response of individual patients to pharmacological treatment.

A similar baseline pattern of high ventral anterior cingulate cortex metabolism predicted response in unipolar depressed patients to treatment with sleep deprivation. Wu and colleagues (1999) (see also the review by Wu et al. 2001) found that high baseline ventral anterior cingulate cortex metabolic values also predicted clinical response in unipolar depressed patients who were treated with sleep deprivation. These researchers studied 36 patients with unipolar depression and 26 nondepressed volunteers with FDG PET before and after sleep deprivation. The authors reported that the depressed subjects who responded to sleep deprivation had higher baseline glucose metabolism in the medial prefrontal cortex, the ventral anterior cingulate cortex, and the posterior subcallosal gyrus than did depressed nonresponders. After sleep deprivation the ventral anterior cingulate cortex metabolism normalized in the responders. These findings give further weight to the involvement of ventral anterior cingulum in response to treatment in unipolar depressed patients, whereas the caudate nucleus appears to have greater importance in treatment response in OCD patients.

Receptor/Transporter Findings in Depression

Because SSRIs are important antidepressants, it is natural to examine the occupancy of the serotonin transporter protein before and after clinical treatment with an SSRI. Meyer et al. (2001) examined occupancy of serotonin transporters in depressed patients after completion of a 6-week trial of either paroxetine or citalopram. The researchers examined 13 unipolar depressed individuals and 17 healthy control subjects. Serotonin transporter (5-HTT) binding was determined with PET and the tracer *N,N*-dimethyl-2-(2-amino-4-cyanophenylthio)benzylamine C 11 at baseline (at least 2 months after discontinuation of antidepressant medication) for the depressed subjects and after 4 weeks of clinical treatment. The authors found no difference in striatal 5-HTT binding potential between control subjects and patients at baseline. They further found that patients treated with 20 mg of paroxetine or 20 mg of citalopram had a mean proportion of occupied 5-HTT sites of roughly 80%. The researchers found no relationship between the final score on the Hamilton Rating Scale for Depression and the 5-HTT occupancy of the striatum. Although reuptake inhibition of 5-HTT is an important method of treatment, the degree of transporter binding in the striatum did not directly correlate with the antidepressant response. The 5-HTT sites occupied in the frontal cortex might have been of interest. Alternatively, physiological changes due to pharmacological treatment that may also occur at another locus farther downstream from transporter binding by the antidepressant might more directly reflect the degree of clinical response.

One location downstream from the transporter is the serotonin receptor. Yatham and colleagues (1999) examined serotonin receptor binding in patients with major depression at baseline and after 3–4 weeks of clinical treatment with desipramine. This paired study was performed with PET and the tracer setoperone F 18. The authors found that cortical 5-HT_2 receptors decreased significantly throughout the cortex after treatment; the decrease was most pronounced in the frontal cortex. The authors noted that it is unknown whether the change in 5-HT_2 receptors is due to clinical improvement or an effect of desipramine unrelated to clinical status. Of the 10 patients in this paired study, 8 (80%) responded to treatment as indicated by a drop of more than 50% in scores on the Hamilton Rating Scale for Depression. Examining familial depression might further enhance the ability to appreciate treatment mechanisms.

Summary

One of the great hopes was that PET would help to increase the understanding of both the underlying pathophysiology of different neuropsychiatric disorders and pharmacological effects on brain function. Such knowledge could help discern which patients would be most likely to respond to pharmacological treatment. Significant progress has been made, but this goal still remains distant.

Conclusion

Imaging techniques have contributed to significant advances in the understanding of the structure and function of the human brain. Improvements in MRI have included not just enhanced resolution and contrast, but also new techniques such as spectroscopy and diffusion tensor imaging, both of which have clinical and research importance. Advances in PET techniques have progressed beyond the measurement of regional glucose metabolism, regional cerebral blood flow, and dopamine receptors to include the imaging of vesicular transporters in monoamine neurons (Gilman et al. 1998). Such developments will continue to help clinicians understand the pathophysiology of neuropsychiatric disorders and the mechanism of action of pharmacological treatments.

Currently, for a given psychiatric disorder such as schizophrenia there may be certain patterns of magnetic resonance or functional abnormalities. However, with current techniques these patterns are not diagnostic for a given subject, nor are they predictive of the subjects' response to treatment. Two directions of development are foreseen. One direction involves the continued development of radioligands that are able to elucidate physiological processes at a finer level, such as imaging molecular genetic processes. Another direction is suggested in the review by Weinberger et al. (2001), in which they note that the catechol-*O*-methyl transferase genotype predicts prefrontal physiology during a working memory task. The incorporation of genetic information into imaging and cognitive studies will perhaps be the more important direction. In general, the study of susceptibility alleles involving, for example, dopaminergic or serotonergic systems in conjunction with neuroimaging studies may eventually lead to diagnostic and treatment information for certain individuals with a neuropsychiatric disorder. In other fields such as mathematics, exciting developments have occurred when techniques and ideas from different fields were amalgamated to solve problems. We expect the same excitement in psychiatric research as ideas from genetics, neuroimaging, and cognitive science collide.

References

Adalsteinsson E, Sullivan E, Kleinhans N, et al: Longitudinal decline of the neuronal marker N-acetyl aspartate in Alzheimer's disease. Lancet 355:1696–1697, 2000

Alexopoulos GS, Kiosses DN, Choi SJ, et al: Frontal white matter microstructure and treatment response of late-life depression: a preliminary study. Am J Psychiatry 159:1929–1932, 2002

American Psychiatric Association: Diagnostic and Statistical Manual of Mental Disorders, 4th Edition. Washington, DC, American Psychiatric Association, 1994

Aylward EH, Harris GJ, Hoehn-Saric R, et al: Normal caudate nucleus in obsessive-compulsive disorder assessed by quantitative neuroimaging. Arch Gen Psychiatry 53:577–584, 1996

Bartha R, Stein MB, Williamson PC, et al: A short echo H-2 spectroscopy and volumetric MRI study of the corpus striatum in patients with obsessive-compulsive disorder and comparison subjects. Am J Psychiatry 155:1584–1591, 1998

Bartha R, Al-Semaan YM, Williamson PC, et al: A short echo proton magnetic resonance spectroscopy study of the left mesial-temporal lobe in first-onset schizophrenic patients. Biol Psychiatry 45:1403–1411, 1999

Baxter LR Jr, Phelps ME, Mazziotta JC, et al: Local cerebral glucose metabolic rates in obsessive-compulsive disorder. A comparison with rates in unipolar depression and in normal controls. Arch Gen Psychiatry 44:211–218, 1987

Baxter LR Jr, Schwartz JM, Bergman KS, et al: Caudate glucose metabolic rate changes with both drug and behavior therapy for obsessive-compulsive disorder. Arch Gen Psychiatry 49:681–689, 1992

Benkelfat C, Nordahl TE, Semple WE, et al: Local cerebral glucose metabolic rates in obsessive-compulsive disorder. Patients treated with clomipramine. Arch Gen Psychiatry 47:840–848, 1990

Bertolino A, Callicot JH, Elman I, et al: Regionally specific neuronal pathology in untreated patients with schizophrenia: a proton magnetic resonance spectroscopic imaging study. Biol Psychiatry 43:641–648, 1998

Bertolino A, Knable MB, Saunders RC, et al: The relationship between dorsolateral prefrontal N-acetylaspartate measures and striatal dopamine activity in schizophrenia. Biol Psychiatry 45:660–667, 1999

Bertolino A, Callicot JH, Mattay VS, et al: The effect of treatment with antipsychotic drugs on brain N-acetylaspartate measures inpatients with schizophrenia. Biol Psychiatry 49:39–46, 2001

Braus DF, Ende G, Weber-Fahr W, et al: Functioning and neuronal viability of the anterior cingulate neurons following antipsychotic treatment: MR-spectroscopic imaging in chronic schizophrenia. Eur Neuropsychopharmacol 12:145–152, 2002

Breier A, Su TP, Saunders R, et al: Schizophrenia is associated with elevated amphetamine-induced synaptic dopamine concentrations: evidence from a novel positron emission tomography method. Proc Natl Acad Sci U S A 94:2569–2574, 1997

Brody AL, Barsom MW, Bota RG, et al: Prefrontal-subcortical and limbic circuit mediation of major depressive disorder. Semin Clin Neuropsychiatry 6:102–112, 2001

Brooks WM, Hodde-Vargas J, Vargas LA, et al: Frontal lobe of children with schizophrenia spectrum disorders: a proton magnetic resonance spectroscopic study. Biol Psychiatry 43:263–269, 1998

Bruhn H, Frahm J, Gyngell ML, et al: Cerebral metabolism in man after acute stroke: new observations using localized proton NMR spectroscopy. Magn Reson Med 9:126–131, 1989

Buchsbaum MS, Ingvar DH, Kessler R, et al: Cerebral glucography with positron tomography: use in normal subjects and in patients with schizophrenia. Arch Gen Psychiatry 39:251–259, 1982

Buchsbaum MS, Potkin SG, Siegel BV Jr, et al: Striatal metabolic rate and clinical response to neuroleptics in schizophrenia. Arch Gen Psychiatry 49:966–974, 1992

Buchsbaum MS, Tang CY, Peled S, et al: MRI white matter diffusion anisotropy and PET metabolic rate in schizophrenia. Neuroreport 9:425–430, 1998

Buckley PF, Moore C, Long H, et al: H-1 magnetic resonance spectroscopy of the left temporal and frontal lobes in schizophrenia: clinical, neurodevelopmental, and cognitive correlates. Biol Psychiatry 36: 792–800, 1994

Bustillo JR, Lauriello J, Rowland LM, et al: Effects of chronic haloperidol and clozapine treatments on frontal and caudate neurochemistry in schizophrenia. Psychiatry Res 107:135–149, 2001

Cabeza R, Nyberg L: Imaging cognition, II: an empirical review of 275 PET and fMRI studies. J Cogn Neurosci 12:1–47, 2000

Chang L, Miller BL, McBride D, et al: Brain lesions in patients with AIDS: H-1 MR spectroscopy. Radiology 197:527–531, 1995

Charles HC, Lazeyras F, Krishnan RR, et al: Brain choline in depression: in vivo detection of potential pharmacodynamic effects of antidepressant therapy using hydrogen localized spectroscopy. Prog Neuropsychopharmacol Biol Psychiatry 18:1121–1127, 1994

Cecil KM, Lenkinski RE, Gur RE, et al: Proton magnetic resonance spectroscopy in the frontal and temporal lobes of neuroleptic naive patients with schizophrenia. Neuropsychopharmacology 20:131–140, 1999

Cohen RM, Nordahl TE, Semple WE, et al: Abnormalities in the distributed network of sustained attention predict neuroleptic treatment response in schizophrenia. Neuropsychopharmacology 19:36–47, 1998

Corson PW, Nopoulos P, Miller DD, et al: Change in basal ganglia volume over 2 years in patients with schizophrenia: typical versus atypical neuroleptics. Am J Psychiatry 156:1200–1204, 1999

Deicken RF, Calabrese G, Merrin EL, et al: ^{31}Phosphorus magnetic resonance spectroscopy of the frontal and parietal lobes in chronic schizophrenia. Biol Psychiatry 36:503–510, 1994

Deicken RF, Zhou L, Corwin F, et al: Decreased left frontal lobe N-acetylaspartate in schizophrenia. Am J Psychiatry 154:688–690, 1997a

Deicken RF, Zhou L, Schuff N, et al: Proton magnetic resonance spectroscopy of the anterior cingulate region in schizophrenia. Schizophr Res 27:65–71, 1997b

Deicken RF, Zhou L, Schuff N, et al: Hippocampal neuronal dysfunction in schizophrenia as measured by proton magnetic resonance spectroscopy. Biol Psychiatry 43:483–488, 1998

de Leon J, Becona E, Gurpegui M, et al: The association between high nicotine dependence and severe mental illness may be consistent across countries. J Clin Psychiatry 63:812–816, 2002

Dumoulin CL, Hart HR Jr: Magnetic resonance angiography. Radiology 161:717–720, 1986

Ebert D, Speck O, Konig A, et al: H-1 magnetic resonance spectroscopy in obsessive-compulsive disorder: evidence for neuronal loss in the cingulate gyrus and the right striatum. Psychiatry Res 74:173–176, 1997

Elkis H, Friedman L, Wise A, et al: Meta-analyses of studies of ventricular enlargement and cortical sulcal prominence in mood disorders: comparisons with controls or patients with schizophrenia. Arch Gen Psychiatry 52:735–746, 1995

Ende GR, Laxer KD, Knowlton RC, et al: Temporal lobe epilepsy: bilateral hippocampal metabolite changes revealed at proton MR spectroscopic imaging. Radiology 202:809–817, 1997

Farde L, Wiesel FA, Nordstrom AL, et al: D1- and D2-dopamine receptor occupancy during treatment with conventional and atypical neuroleptics. Psychopharmacology 99:S28–S31, 1989

Farde L, Nyberg S, Oxenstierna G, et al: Positron emission tomography studies on D2 and 5-HT2 receptor binding in risperidone-treated schizophrenic patients. J Clin Psychopharmacol 15:19S–23S, 1995

Feinberg I: Cortical pruning and the development of schizophrenia. Schizophr Bull 16:567–570, 1990

Foong J, Symms MR, Barker GJ, et al: Investigating regional white matter in schizophrenia using diffusion tensor imaging. Neuroreport 13:333–336, 2002

Fowler JS, Volkow ND, Wang G-J, et al: Brain monoamine oxidase A inhibition in cigarette smokers. Proc Natl Acad Sci U S A 93:14065–14069,1996a

Fowler JS, Volkow ND, Wang G-J, et al: Inhibition of monoamine oxidase B in the brains of smokers. Nature 379:733–736, 1996b

Friedman SD, Brooks WM, Jung RE, et al: Quantitative proton predicts outcome after traumatic brain injury. Neurology 52:1384–1391, 1999

Giedd JN, Jeffries NO, Blumenthal J, et al: Childhood-onset schizophrenia: progressive brain changes during adolescence. Biol Psychiatry 46:892–898, 1999

Gilman S, Koeppe RA, Adams KM, et al: Decreased striatal monoaminergic terminals in severe chronic alcoholism demonstrated with (1)[11C]dihydrotetrabenazine and positron emission tomography. Ann Neurol 44:326–333, 1998

Gonen O, Catalaa I, Babb JS, et al: Total brain N-acetylaspartate: a new measure of disease load in MS. Neurology 54:15–19, 2000

Gur RE, Mozley PD, Resnick SM, et al: Resting cerebral glucose metabolism in first-episode and previously treated patients with schizophrenia relates to clinical features. Arch Gen Psychiatry 52:657–667, 1995

Hietala J, Synalahti E, Vuorio K, et al: Striatal D2-dopamine receptor characteristics in neuroleptic-naïve schizophrenic patients studied with positron emission tomography. Arch Gen Psychiatry 51:116–123, 1994

Ingvar D, Franzen G: Distribution of cerebral activity in chronic schizophrenia. Lancet 2:1484–1486, 1974

Kapur S, Seeman P: Does fast dissociation from the dopamine D-2 receptor explain the action of atypical antipsychotics?: a new hypothesis. Am J Psychiatry 158:360–369, 2001

Ketter TA, George MS, Kimbrell TA, et al: Functional brain imaging, limbic function, and affective disorders. Neuroscientist 2:55–65, 1996

Kubicki M, Westin CF, Maier SE, et al: Uncinate fasciculus findings in schizophrenia: a diffusion tensor imaging study. Am J Psychiatry 159:813–820, 2002

Laruelle M, Abi-Dargham A, van Dyck CH, et al: Single photon emission computerized tomography imaging of amphetamine-induced dopamine release in drug-free schizophrenic subjects. Proc Natl Acad Sci U S A 93:9235–9240, 1996

Lawrie SM, Whalley H, Kestelman JN, et al: Magnetic resonance imaging of brain in people at high risk of developing schizophrenia. Lancet 353:30–33, 1999

Lim KO, Tew W, Kushner M, et al: Cortical gray matter volume deficit in patients with first-episode schizophrenia. Am J Psychiatry 153:1548–1553, 1996

Lim KO, Adalsteinsson E, Spielman D, et al: Proton magnetic resonance spectroscopic imaging of cortical gray and white matter in schizophrenia. Arch Gen Psychiatry 55:346–352, 1998

Lim KO, Hedehus M, Moseley M, et al: Compromised white matter tract integrity in schizophrenia inferred from diffusion tensor imaging. Arch Gen Psychiatry 56:367–374, 1999

Mayberg HS, Brannan SK, Mahurin RK, et al: Cingulate function in depression: a potential predictor of treatment response. Neuroreport 8:1057–1061, 1997

Meltzer HY, Matsubara S, Lee JC: Classification of typical and atypical antipsychotic drugs on the basis of dopamine D1, D2, and serotonin2 pKi values. J Pharmacol Exp Ther 251:238–246, 1989

Meyer JH, Wilson AA, Ginovart N, et al: Occupancy of serotonin transporters by paroxetine and citalopram during treatment of depression: a [(11)C]DASB PET imaging study. Am J Psychiatry 158:1843–1849, 2001

Nasrallah HA, Skinner TE, Schmalbrock P, et al: Proton magnetic resonance spectroscopy of the hippocampal formation in schizophrenia: a pilot study. Br J Psychiatry 165:481–485, 1994

Nordahl TE, Benkelfat C, Semple WE, et al: Cerebral glucose metabolic rates in obsessive compulsive disorder. Neuropsychopharmacology 2:23–28, 1989

Nordahl TE, Carter CS, Salo RS, et al: Anterior cingulate metabolism correlates with Stroop errors in paranoid schizophrenia patients. Neuropsychopharmacology 25:139–148, 2001

Patterson JC II, Kotrla KJ: Functional neuroimaging in psychiatry, in The American Psychiatric Publishing Textbook of Neuropsychiatry and Clinical Neurosciences, 4th Edition. Edited by Yudofsky SC, Hales RE. Washington, DC, American Psychiatric Publishing, 2002, pp 285–321

Perani D, Colombo C, Bressi S, et al: 18-FDG PET study in obsessive-compulsive disorder. A clinical/metabolic correlation study after treatment. Br J Psychiatry 166:244–250, 1995

Pfefferbaum A, Adalsteinsson A, Spielman D, et al: In vivo brain concentrations of N-acetyl compounds, creatine and choline in Alzheimer's disease. Arch Gen Psychiatry 56:185–192, 1999

Pfefferbaum A, Sullivan EV, Hedehus M, et al: Age-related decline in brain white matter anisotropy measured with spatially corrected echo-planar diffusion tensor imaging. Magn Reson Med 44:259–268, 2000

Pierpaoli C, Basser PJ: Toward a quantitative assessment of diffusion anisotropy. Magn Reson Med 36:893–906, 1996 [erratum in Magn Reson Med 37:972, 1997]

Renshaw PF, Parow AM, Hirashima F, et al: Multinuclear magnetic resonance spectroscopy studies of brain purines in major depression. Am J Psychiatry 158:2048–2055, 2001
Rogers MA, Bradshaw JL, Pantelis C, et al: Frontostriatal deficits in unipolar major depression. Brain Res Bull 47:297–310, 1998
Saxena S, Brody AL, Ho ML, et al: Differential brain metabolic predictors of response to paroxetine in obsessive-compulsive disorder versus major depression. Am J Psychiatry 160:522–532, 2003
Schweinsburg BC, Taylor MJ, Alhassoon OM, et al: Chemical pathology in brain white matter of recently detoxified alcoholics: a 1H magnetic resonance spectroscopy investigation of alcohol-associated frontal lobe injury. Alcohol Clin Exp Res 25:924–934, 2001
Seeman P, Bzowej NH, Guan HC, et al: Human brain D1 and D2 dopamine receptors in schizophrenia, Alzheimer's, Parkinson's, and Huntington's diseases. Neuropsychopharmacology 1:5–15, 1987
Sharma T, Lancaster E, Sigmundsson T, et al: Lack of normal pattern of cerebral asymmetry in familial schizophrenic patients and their relatives—The Maudsley Family Study. Schizophr Res 40:111–120, 1999
Shenton ME, Dickey CC, Frumin M, et al: A review of MRI findings in schizophrenia. Schizophr Res 49:1–52, 2001
Steel RM, Bastin ME, McConnell S, et al: Diffusion tensor imaging (DTI) and proton magnetic resonance spectroscopy (1H MRS) in schizophrenic subjects and normal controls. Psychiatry Res 106:161–170, 2001
Swedo SE, Schapiro MB, Grady CL, et al: Cerebral glucose metabolism in childhood-onset obsessive-compulsive disorder. Arch Gen Psychiatry 46:518–523, 1989
Swedo SE, Pietrini P, Leonare HL, et al: Cerebral glucose metabolism in childhood-onset obsessive-compulsive disorder: revisualization during pharmacotherapy. Arch Gen Psychiatry 49:690–694, 1992
Tamminga CA, Thaker GK, Buchanan R, et al: Limbic system abnormalities identified in schizophrenia using positron emission tomography with fluorodeoxyglucose and neocortical alterations with deficit syndrome. Arch Gen Psychiatry 49:522–530, 1992
Taylor WD, Payne ME, Krishnan KR, et al: Evidence of white matter tract disruption in MRI hyperintensities. Biol Psychiatry 50:179–183, 2001
Tsai G, Coyle JT: N-acetylaspartate in neuropsychiatric disorders. Prog Neurobiol 46:531–540, 1995
Valk PE, Dillon WP: Radiation injury of the brain. AJNR Am J Neuroradiol 12:45–62, 1991

Videbech P: MRI findings in patients with affective disorder: a meta-analysis. Acta Psychiatr Scand 96:157–168, 1997

Volkow ND, Brodie JD, Wolf AP, et al: Brain metabolism in patients with schizophrenia before and after acute neuroleptic administration. J Neurol Neurosurg Psychiatry 49:1199–1202, 1986

Wagner HN, Burns HD, Dannals RF, et al: Imaging dopamine receptors in the human brain by positron tomography. Science 221:1264–1266, 1983

Weinberger DR, Egan MF, Bertolino A, et al: Neurobiology of schizophrenia and the role of atypical antipsychotics prefrontal neurons and the genetics of schizophrenia. Biol Psychiatry 50:825–844, 2001

Wolkin A, Jaeger J, Brodie JD, et al: Persistence of cerebral metabolic abnormalities in chronic schizophrenia as determined by positron emission tomography. Am J Psychiatry 142:564–571, 1985

Wolkin A, Choi SJ, Szilagyi S, et al: Inferior frontal white matter anisotropy and negative symptoms of schizophrenia: a diffusion tensor imaging study. Am J Psychiatry 160:572–574, 2003

Wu J, Buchsbaum MS, Gillin JC, et al: Predictions of antidepressant effects of sleep deprivation by metabolic rates in the ventral anterior cingulate and medial prefrontal cortex. Am J Psychiatry 156:1149–1158, 1999

Wu JC, Buchsbaum M, Bunney W Jr: Clinical neurochemical implications of sleep deprivation's effects on the anterior cingulate of depressed responders. Neuropsychopharmacology 25 (suppl 5):S74–S78, 2001

Yatham LN, Liddle PF, Dennie J, et al: Decrease in brain serotonin 2 receptor binding in patients with major depression following desipramine treatment: a positron emission tomography study with fluorine-18 labeled setoperone. Arch Gen Psychiatry 56:705–711, 1999

Yurgelun-Todd DA, Renshaw PF, Gruber SA, et al: Proton magnetic resonance spectroscopy of the temporal lobes in schizophrenics and normal controls. Schizophr Res 19:55–59, 1996

Afterword

Stuart C. Yudofsky, M.D.
H. Florence Kim, M.D.

The human brain is thought to be the most complex entity in the observable universe, and its most intricate and relevant functions involve memory, cognition, mood regulation, and impulse regulation. For millennia, brain-based dysfunctions in memory, cognition, mood and impulse regulation have been accepted as unfortunate "realities" of the human condition, far beyond man's ability to understand, treat or prevent. Over the last decade, however, advances in key areas of basic and laboratory science—including molecular biology, cell biology, genetics, neuroscience, neuropathology and neuroimaging—have helped to establish new and meaningful links between neurobiologic abnormalities and neuropsychiatric disorders. The opportunities for translational research in these realms are robust, so we can expect important innovations in our abilities to diagnose and treat—with greater specificity and safety—people with neuropsychiatric conditions. We fully expect that the neuropsychiatric assessment will remain an essential and integrating body of knowledge and skills that is requisite to take full advantage of the revolutionary advances in neurobiology in the diagnosis and treatment of the many people with neuropsychiatric disorders. In this small volume, we have endeavored to provide a useful update.

Index

Page numbers printed in ***boldface*** *type refer to tables or figures.*